MW00459851

A Brief History of Yoga

From Its Tantric Roots to the Modern Yoga Studio

By The Same Author

Sacred Body, Sacred Spirit
Principles for a Balanced Economy
Tantra: The Yoga of Love and Awakening
Growing a New Economy

A Brief History of Yoga

From Its Tantric Roots to the Modern Yoga Studio

Ramesh Bjonnes

InnerWorld Publications
San Germán, Puerto Rico
www.innerworldpublications.com

Copyright © 2018 by Ramesh Bjonnes

All rights reserved under International and Pan-American Copyright Conventions. Published in the United States by InnerWorld Publications, PO Box 1613, San Germán, Puerto Rico, 00683.

Library of Congress Catalog Card Number: 2018947206

Cover Design © Aaron Ananta Staengl

No part of this book may be reproduced or transmitted in any form or by any means, electronic or mechanical, including photocopying, recording, or by any information storage or retrieval system, without permission in writing from the publisher, except for the inclusion of brief quotations in a review.

ISBN 9781881717638

Contents

Introduction   1

Chapter One
Yoga, Tantra and the Vedas   20

Chapter Two
The Union of Tantra and Yoga   26

Chapter Three
A Brief Tantric History of Yoga   51

Chapter Four
Dravidians and Aryans:
Cultural Clash and Integration   72

Chapter Five
The Path of Union:
The Philosophy and Practice of Tantric Yoga   100

Bibliography   136

Glossary   140

Introduction

MOST AUTHORS WRITING ABOUT yoga history have claimed that yoga originated in the Vedas. In recent years, however, some Western yoga scholars have begun to question this view, including James Mallinson and Mark Singleton, authors of the monumental book *Roots of Yoga*. Although they acknowledge that many aspects of Vedic society reflect the yoga tradition to some extent, they emphasize that the practice and culture of yoga originated outside the Vedic tradition. Likewise, in India, many writers and teachers of yoga have long pointed out that the tradition has deep historical roots in the soil of Shaivism, more popularly known as Tantra.

In the early 1980s, when I lived in an Ashram in Nepal studying and practicing Tantra, I began to understand the complex historical reasons why the real roots of yoga had remained hidden for so long. It all began when a Nepali friend simply wanted to learn the practice of Tantric yoga.

When I was not studying and practicing yoga and meditation in the ashram, my job was to shop for vegetables, fruits and rice in an outdoor market near the ashram. During one of those shopping trips, I made friends with a young Nepali Brahmin whose face brightened with excitement every time I told him stories about my guru and about Tantra and yoga. During one of those shopping trips, he told me that he wanted to learn Tantric meditation.

Since traditional Tantra does not accept the caste system, I told him he had to renounce his allegiance to his Brahmin social status in order to be initiated. He had to both literally and symbolically cut the white cotton thread marking him as an upper-caste Hindu. Upon hearing that, he hesitated at first, but since he was young and adventurous, a few weeks later, he decided to take the leap into the new and enigmatic world of yoga and Tantra.

For several weeks after the initiation, my friend visited the ashram almost daily to meditate and to practice yoga postures with us. Judging from his relaxed and friendly demeanor, it was obvious he enjoyed his new practice and lifestyle. I was therefore very surprised when one day, without notice, he suddenly stopped visiting us. A few weeks later, one of the shopkeepers at the market told me the young man's uncle had forced him to return to the family village. "They became angry when they heard he had renounced his caste," the shopkeeper said.

Back in the village, my friend's father threatened him with banishment from the family "unless he put the Brahmin thread back on." Instead of breaking with family tradition and religious dogma, he complied with his father's stern ultimatum, and he never returned to the ashram to practice Tantric yoga again.

Discrimination and division based on caste has been illegal in India since the 1940s, but the caste system is still vibrantly alive, especially in marriage and in politics. A 2014 survey by the Indian National Council of Economic Research found that almost 1/3 of all Indians still would not admit a person from the Dalit community (a so-called untouchable or casteless) into their kitchen or to use their utensils. Very few marry outside their caste, even today, and most people vote for politicians based on his or her caste. The ancient hierarchy of caste—which makes Brahmins (priests and teachers), Ksyattrias (warriors) and Vyashyas (merchants) superior to the Shudras (workers), not to speak of the Dalits —has been part of Indian society since the beginning of historical time, since the arrival of the Vedic Aryans, who gradually solidified the rigors of caste, first in the Vedas, then in the Manusmriti, a Hindu text on morals, traditions and caste. The Manusmriti prevents widows to remarry and Brahmin men to marry a woman of a lower caste. But what does all this have to do with the history of yoga? As we shall soon learn, quite a lot.

Some scholars and teachers of the yoga tradition have always pointed out that Tantra, and therefore, they claim, yoga developed outside of Brahmin society, largely beyond the dogmas and influences of priestly rituals. As a spiritual tradition, Tantra has therefore both been an influential and a subversive force in Indian culture, both despised and admired as a religion, both feared and embraced as a culture of the poor. Since yoga and Tantra originally developed outside the dominance of the Vedic Brahmins, mostly among the Shudras and the casteless, the real story of where, how and when yoga originated, the people's history of yoga, if you will, has largely been overlooked by Western academics and historians, as well as by most Indian writers. This book is my attempt at telling the story of yoga from the point of view of Tantra—which some scholars call "the people's religion" of India. This book is my attempt at presenting why and how Tantra, more than the Veda, is the main source of yoga, its history, practice and philosophy.

The Two Branches of Yoga:
The Vedic and the Tantric

How old is yoga? Who invented its meditation and posture practices? Scholars and practitioners have been trying to answer these questions for many years, and there are currently both conflicting and overlapping views on how and when yoga emerged. Until recently, the majority of Western scholars traced the early roots of yoga to the ancient Vedas, most notably to the Rigveda and the Atharvaveda. Recent scholarship, as well as the Puranas and the contemporary writings of Tantric master Anandamurtii, has shown that yoga originated outside the Vedic tradition, among the ancient Shaiva Tantrics. This tradition is generally referred to as "the parallel tradition" in relation to the Vedas. It is now believed, however, that many early Vedic texts absorbed Tantric ideas, making it seem as if yoga originated in the Vedic texts, while the actual origin was Tantra. Likewise, Buddhist and Jain texts were also greatly influenced by Tantra.

There are four Vedic texts—the Rigveda, the Atharvaveda, the Samaveda and the Yajurveda. The first and oldest text, the Rigveda was, according to B.G. Sidharth and others, composed outside India by Vedic Aryan priests, in a patriarchal society, as early as perhaps 12,000 BCE. The other three texts were mostly composed inside India and influenced by the Tantric tradition and the indigenous peoples to various degrees. (Sidharth, 1999). As these Vedas were composed over time, first as oral *sutras* and much later as written texts, there was a gradual sophistication in their philosophical expression. This sophistication blossomed especially in the Upanishads and the Brahmanas, texts which are sometimes termed the Fifth Veda and which later developed into the philosophical system of Vedanta. These Vedic texts, however, were also greatly influenced by the Shaiva yogis. In fact, the sophisticated spiritual insights composed in these texts were inspired by people who practiced yogic or Tantric meditation rather than priestly Vedic rituals. Later on, in the Middle Ages, when the Tantric teachings, such as the ancient sutras from the Agamas, were written down, yoga philosophy was given a distinct Tantric flavor. (Anandamurtii, 1993)

There have been largely two predominant archetypes of religion throughout history: the priest and the mystic—the priest as interpreter and believer, the mystic as practitioner and union-with-the-Divine seeker. In India, these two archetypes are represented by the Vedic priest and the Tantric yogi. The priests were always male, the yogis were mostly male but also female. The priest mostly engaged in various chants and rituals, the yogi engaged, first in shamanic practices, then in disciplined contemplation, physical and mental exercises to experience union with the inner and outer universe. The priests were mostly Vedic Aryans at first, the yogis were mostly indigenous Dravidians, Mongolians and Austrics (the first inhabitants of India). Over time, the lines between priest and yogi, between the invading Aryans and the indigenous peoples became blurred, sometimes a priest also turned yogi; but yogis most often remained yogis while adopting some of the rituals and chants of the priests. Over time, India became a blended civilization, and by the time the Tantras were written down in the Middle Ages, only the learned few could distinguish what was original Tantric yoga and what had been influenced by the Brahmanic culture of the Vedic people (Anandamurtii, 1993).

By the time the first Upanishads were written around 500 BCE, the Vedic and Tantric cultures had merged to such an extent that it was common that some Brahmin priests, in addition to their sacrificial fire rituals also practiced Tantric meditation (Ananadamurtii, 1993). The Vedic and yogic texts, which were written several thousand years after the yogic tradition developed, were thus written in a blended society, where both Vedic rituals and Tantric yoga practices co-existed and formed a new civilization, today better known as the Indian or the Hindu civilization.

From the confluence of these two rivers, the Vedic and the Tantric, yoga developed during a complex, long, colorful and sometimes violent history spanning perhaps over 7000 years. Of these two rivers of religion and wisdom, the Shaiva Tantric stream has shaped the tradition of yoga the most (Bhattacharyya, 1982). As Anandamurtii writes in his essay Tantra and Indo-Aryan Civilization: "From the non-Aryans the Aryans acquired a well-knit social system, a subtle insight, spiritual philosophy and Tantra *sadhana* [yoga practices]." (Anandamurtii, 1993)

Sources and Methods of Inquiry

During the writing of this book, I have relied almost exclusively on English translations of Sanskrit texts from the original, on numerous books about yoga, Tantra and Indian history, on research in archeology and genetics, on the personal accounts of teachers and practitioners, on the latest scholarship in yoga history, as well as the writings of gurus within the Tantra tradition, especially the writings of Anandamurtii, who introduced new aspects of Tantra philosophy and practice and made unorthodox statements about yoga history, some of which have been confirmed by science, others which are yet to be ratified. For a detailed list of source materials, please consult the bibliography at the end of the book.

In writings about history, it is common to rely on textual documentation, archeology, etc., in order to draw conclusions. In other words, the scientific method of study is most commonly applied to determine facts, timelines, etc. as it is considered the most objective and unbiased way of receiving information. However, no method of knowing is without limitations, including the scientific method. Observable data takes on meanings that may be interpreted in a biased fashion. Objective information may mask important subjective influences, and not all phenomena are easily observable. Moreover, as new data becomes available old scientific opinions are overturned. Therefore, I have not only relied on texts and studied the history in an academic fashion, but also consulted other ways of knowing that may be relevant to creating a broader and thus more comprehensive portrait of the history of yoga.

The Four Ways of Knowing

According to the epistemology of Samkhya, the oldest system of Indian philosophy, there are three valid ways of knowing the real: 1) perception or empiricism; 2) inference or logic; 3) testimony or authority. There is also a fourth way of knowing according to yogic epistemology, namely intuition. In this book, I have relied on all of these ways of knowing to gather data, explanations, quotes and insights about the complex history of India in general and yoga in particular. Rather than relying on academic information and scientific methods of gathering data, which is the main method of Western academia, I have, in the spirit of yoga, also relied on the testimony of great masters of yoga as well as their intuitive wisdom. These four ways of knowing—empiricism, logic, authority, and intuition—are all valid ways to shape our understanding of reality, but, as noted below, with each way of knowing there are also potential shortcomings:

Empiricism or science. Empirical knowledge is grounded in facts and science, such as in dating texts or an archeological find. One limitation of scientific inquiry, however, is that all artifacts are observed and interpreted by subjective minds and information gathered may therefore be biased. As an example, a significant artifact in yoga history is the Pashupatinat seal (Marshall, 1928), an alleged yogic deity, perhaps linked to Shiva, surrounded by animals. Archeologist John Marshall named the seal Pashupatinat, because Shiva is considered the protector of animals (pashu), and because the yogi is a controller of his or her animal instincts. This seal has been quite accurately dated to about 2300 BCE. It is also quite clear to the majority of scholars that the person on the seal sits in a yogic *asana*, or posture, but to be absolutely certain about who the figure is or represents is not so easy. But other ways of knowing—logic, authority and intuition—may help shed more light on what this figure represents. Naturally, there are several conflicting views on what this seal signifies. Similarly, texts can often be accurately dated but the meaning of the texts, who its writers were, what the religious sources are, and so on, can often be up for interpretation. It is an empirical fact that there are many references to Tantra in certain portions of the Atharvaveda. This has led some scholars to claim that these teachings are Vedic. An authoritative Tantric source, such as Anandamurtii, points out, however, that these passages were appropriated from Tantric teachings and included in this Vedic text. Several Indologists have made similar claims. The scientific method alone is therefore not always enough to accurately verify certain "facts."

Logic and reason. This kind of knowledge does not depend on sensory information but rather on logic, internal consistency and common sense. Philosophical knowledge is often judged by logic and reason, such as is often done when comparing the yoga philosophy of Patanjali to that of Kapila's Samkhya, or when Tantra is compared to Vedanta, or when a Vedic text supposedly contains not commonly known or "hidden" Tantric passages. When looking at all the scholarly comments about the Pashupatinat seal and what it could represent, Indologist Doris Meth Srinivasanwrote in a 1976 article, otherwise critical of Marshall's interpretation, by observing that "no matter what position is taken regarding the seal's iconography, it is always prefaced by Marshall's interpretation. On balance the proto-*Siva*character of the seal has been accepted.» No matter what the figure represents, most scholars agree that the figure sits in a yogic position,. And if the seal indeed represent a yogic or Tantric figure sitting in a position that resembles the *goraksha-asana* position (Feuerstein, 2008), then yoga is much older than what is today commonly accepted. But logical arguments can also be limited. An author may, for example, claim to prove that a passage is Vedic in a Tantric text or vice versa, but this argument may contain logical fallacies or be based on social, cultural or religious biases.

Authority. This form of knowledge utilizes the wisdom of "great" people and traditions, those who have been time-tested through some process of social validation, peer review or by proving they have deep knowledge in a certain field, such as philosophy, the intuitional science of mantra, or in asana practice. Thus many authoritative scholars have concluded that the Pashupatinath figure mentioned above, indeed represents a yogi seated in an advanced yoga position, or asana. Hence, from that information, we may conclude that yoga history is not only 2500 years old (Mallinson and Singleton, 2017) but at least 4500 years old and perhaps 7000 years old or more (Anandamurtii, 1993). In the Indian context, the spiritual authority is the guru, who is respected and judged by his or her wisdom, actions, knowledge of scriptures and intuitional knowledge of the subtle, science of yoga and Tantra. It is therefore accepted in yoga that the teacher is an authority and the upholder of truth, which is both absolute (spiritual) as well as relative (worldly). These savants of the spirit, these Einsteins of consciousness (Hixon, 1978), often display insights and knowledge beyond common perceptions, and these *siddhis*, these psychic abilities, have been experienced by numerous practitioners of yoga (myself included) and are well documented in numerous books about Indian gurus. Their authority is thus often located beyond empirical science, logic and reason. But it is also located in the intellectual realm, in understanding the texts, their origins and influences—how some texts have been influenced by the Vedas and others by the Tantras. In this regard, Anandamurtii and others have pointed out many Tantric influences in the Vedic literature. Mythology and the genealogy of ancient texts, such as the Puranas, which in addition to the Vedas and the Tantras are the three main textual sources in India, may also contain authoritative, historical facts. Anandamurtii refer, for example to Shiva as the source of the various forms of yoga, including a special form termed Rajadhiraja yoga, King of Kings Yoga. This form of yoga is also referred to in the Tantras, the treatises on the magic sciences, as simply Shiva Yoga (Danielou, 1991). This form of Tantric yoga, according to Anandamurtii, specializes in breath yoga with mantras and in practicing special posture yoga exercises to balance the physical and subtle body in preparation for deep meditation. This yoga was revived by Astavakra a few hundred years before Patanjali codified Raja Yoga in the Yoga Sutras, and again modified by Anandamurtii for modern times. If these authorities are correct, then yoga originated with Shiva, some 7000 years ago as Tantra, then developed over time and branched into various forms of Shaiva Tantra, including Hatha Yoga, Laya Yoga, Mantra Yoga, and Rajadhiraja, or Shiva Yoga, and also as various schools of Tantra, including Shakta Tantra, Kashmir Shaivism, Kula Tantra, Vaishnava Tantra, and so on. (Danielou, 1991). But yogic authorities, as well as scientific and philosophical ones, can be wrong, or they may simply represent the popular views of an era, a community of peer reviewers, a sect, or a religious belief. Undivided deference to an authority, whether an academic or a guru, may also hinder our own critical thinking or judgement.

Intuition. The most common understanding of intuition is "a hunch" or "a feeling" but in yoga and Tantra, intuitive knowledge means to have extra-sensory awareness, to have paranormal abilities, to be able to know a person's past, to grasp various subjects without the use of books or Google. Those who have read Swami Yogananda's *Autobiography of a Yogi* or the *Jamalpur Years*, a biography about the early life of Shrii Shrii Ananandamurtii, have learned that great yogis possess these psychic powers of intuition. And within the Indian episteme, these powers are readily accepted since the ultimate truth is beyond, but includes, both mind and matter. The yogis thus claim control and influence over both the psychic and physical realities. Ultimate truth, according to yoga, is beyond the relative truth of the mental and physical world; it resides in Ananda, or bliss, and is achieved when a yogi attains Cosmic Consciousness, or enlightenment. In accordance with Tantric philosophy, Anandamurtii described theuniverseas a result of "macropsychicconation" – that the entire universe exists within the cosmic mind, which itself is the first expression of consciousness coming under the bondage of its own nature. A yogi, in a state of cosmic consciouness thus becomes master and knower of both worlds, the psychic and the physical. And this cosmic state of enlightenment, as many first-hand accounts of disciple stories have testified to, may express itself in the form of clairvoyance or extrasensory perception (ESP), abilities that defy current scientific laws or scrutiny. Gurus may reveal suppressed, as well as known, personal experiences of a disciple as a teaching tool. They may see into the future as well as the past, because their vision is in the ever-present cosmic now, which transcends both future and past, both known psychic and physical realities. This intuitional knowledge is not irrational or unreal, as the sceptics contend, but rather trans-rational, part of a broader science that includes the mental and spiritual domains. Thus Anandamurtii can, through ESP, reconstruct the history of the past and claim that Shiva is the founder of yoga and Tantra, and that both Shiva and Krishna, like the Buddha, were historical figures. The intuitive Anandamurtii wrote, for example, in his book about Shiva, who according to him was the first great master of Tantra, that the Vedic Aryans came into India about 5000 BCE (Anandamurtii, 1983). At the time the book was written, the academic consensus was that the Vedic Aryans migrated to India around 2000 BCE. The new timing of the Aryan migration into India, as suggested by Anandamurtii, was verified by the genetic science of Dr. Spencer Wells and his team a few decades later, even the area from where Anandamurtii said they had originated—the southern steppes of Russia and the Ukraine. Here is an abstract from an online interview with Dr. Wells in 2002:

Interviewer: "Some people say the Aryans are the original inhabitants of India. What is your view on this theory?" Dr. Wells: "The Aryans came from outside India. We actually have genetic evidence for that. Very clear genetic evidence from a marker that arose on the southern steppes of Russia and the Ukraine around 5,000 to 10,000 years ago. And it subsequently spread to the east and south through Central Asia reaching India. It is on the higher frequency in the Indo-European speakers, the people who claim they are descendants of the Aryans, the Hindi speakers, the Bengalis, the other groups. Then it is at a lower frequency in the Dravidians. But there is clear evidence that there was a heavy migration from the steppes down towards India."

Interviewer: "But some people claim that the Aryans were the original inhabitants of India. What do you have to say about this?"

Dr. Wells: "I don't agree with them. The Aryans came later, after the Dravidians." (www.rediff.com, 2002)

For Anandamurtii, yoga is not a religion or a belief system. Neither is yoga anti-science, but rather an "intuitional science," a way of experiencing and interpreting the world where all ways of knowing can harmoniously merge, and a broader, more holistic worldview and science can evolve. If we only rely on intuition, however, and if the seer is not a true sage with extrasensory perception, the intuitive insights may be nothing but a hunch. Indeed, intuition may be guesswork at best, downright wrong at worst, and, as is often the case with religion, can lead to a mythic and dogmatic belief system.

When we take all of these four ways of knowing into account, not only the scientific, academic or textual-based method, but also the philosophies, stories and myths of history as written in the Agamas, the Vedas, the Upanishads, the Puranas, the Bhagavad Gita, the Tantras, etc., as well as the opinions and insights of traditional masters and gurus, I believe that a more comprehensive portrait of yoga history can emerge. This narrative history, which blends the insights of science, rationality, text, and teacher, thus reflect not only the opinions of academia—which generally ignores the historical insights of gurus or independent writers such as Alain Danielou—but also those of the practitioners and the masters. By including a wider range of information, we can hopefully gain a more comprehensive view of the story of yoga. It is my opinion, then, that when we as interpreters of the evolution of yoga embrace a way of knowing the real that is more aligned with the tradition of yoga itself, we can not only comprehend the history of its sciences, logic and authorities, but also the insights of its founders, the great sages, the spiritual custodians of intuition.

The People's History of Yoga

There is a controversial debate going on today about whether the Vedic Aryans migrated to India or not. This debate is riddled with racial, religious and political overtones to such an extent that scientific facts, such as genetic evidence of migration patterns, are often interpreted through the lens of those same racial or religious belief systems. Similarly, the claim that yoga originated in the Vedas is upheld by many as an indisputable truth, while new evidence points toward yoga originating outside the Vedic culture, a claim made not only by academics, but also by gurus and texts within the yogic tradition itself.

Since history is mostly written by the dominant classes, and because the Vedic Aryans have been the predominant power in India for thousands of years, the history of not only India, but also of yoga, has been written from that dominant class' point of view. In addition, the early version of the Aryan Invasion Theory (AIT) was also influenced by the European colonialist mindset of the British and the German scholars, who often stressed that India is great because of the invading Aryans. The Indians today who vehemently oppose the AIT are therefore reacting against this so-called Euro-centric view of India. Which reminds me of a well-known quote from Howard Zinn's monumental book *People's History of the United States*, in which he writes:

"The history of any country, presented as the history of a family, conceals fierce conflicts of interest (sometimes exploding, most often repressed) between conquerors and conquered, masters and slaves, capitalists and workers, dominators and dominated in race and sex. And in such a world of conflict, a world of victims and executioners, it is the job of thinking people, as Albert Camus suggested, not to be on the side of the executioners."

(Zinn, 1980)

This brief book about the history of yoga is an attempt to encourage thinking yogis to take a look at the often untold history of yoga, its hidden past and its many untold stories. This book pays homage to the many known and unknown yogis of the past. It pays tribute to the suppressed history of yoga from the point of view of the conquered, from the point of view of the lower classes and castes, most especially the casteless—the indigenous Shaiva Tantrics, who often defied notions of caste and class and who actually invented yoga, not as a path of ritual and sacrifice, but as a path of liberation and enlightenment.

When we look beyond the cultural, political and sexist biases of history, a new history may emerge—the history of great men and women, who often against all odds, chartered a new path for humanity. The history and practice of yoga, therefore, is not great because of any specific race, but only to the extent that it has empowered and enlightened common people of various races and genders to become liberated agents of their own spiritual destiny.

A New Perspective on the History of Yoga

Using the above four ways of knowing in studying the history of yoga, the following timelines and narratives in yoga history have emerged as some of the most significant:

Posture Yoga (1920 CE): Modern yoga, as practiced in yoga studios worldwide, is a body-centered practice of Hatha Yoga which largely broke with tradition and originated in the 1920s with T. K.V. Krishnamacharya and his school of yoga in Mysore, India. Krishnamacharya and his students claim that his practices are derived from an ancient text titled *Yoga Kuruntha* and his Himalayan guru Yogeshvara Ramamohan Brahmachari, but new research, as documented in the book *Yoga Body* by Mark Singleton, indicate that his system of asana practices is not simply a set of traditional poses but are also combined with Western style gymnastics and poses of his own invention. Modern posture yoga practice as taught in today's yoga studios is a derivation of his style and those resulting from the innovations of his main students, B.K.S. Iyengar, Pattahbi Jois, Indra Devi, and his son T.K.V. Desikachar. Western students of these four trailblazers of modern yoga, including Rodney Yee, Richard Hittleman, Ganga White, and many more, have created modified styles of their own—a tradition which has turned into a multi-billion dollar yoga industry and which continuous to create yet newer styles of posture yoga to this day. Through the practices of posture yoga, a smaller but growing number of students are seeking more traditional forms of yoga by blending Hatha Yoga with more meditative and mystical forms of yoga, including Raja Yoga, Bhakti Yoga, Vedanta and Tantra.

Modernized Traditional Yoga (late 1800s CE): Swami Vivekananda, who arrived in America in 1893, was the first Indian yogi to formulate a modern style of yoga which focused more on meditation and was based on the traditions of Vedanta, Tantra and Raja Yoga. In his footsteps, many other yogis and gurus taught a modern combination of Tantric and Vedantic yoga—teachers such as Swami Yogananda, Swami Muktananada, Swami Satchitananada, Sri Aurobindu, as well as Shrii Shrii Anandamurti. Following in the tradition of Kapila's Samkhya and Patanjali's Yoga Sutras, Anandamurtii composed a new set of Tantra-oriented sutras in a text titled Ananda Sutram.

Traditional Hatha Yoga (500-1500 CE): Yoga as a body-centered practice was popularized in the middle ages through various texts as a form of Tantric Hatha Yoga by legendary teachers such as Matsyendranath and his disciple Goraksanath. Some of these texts, such as Svatmarama's Hatha Yoga Pradipika (1500 CE), also stressed the importance of Raja Yoga, the meditative practices described by Patanajali in the Yoga Sutras, thus emphasizing that yoga is first and foremost a spiritual practice.

Traditional Tantra: (500-1500 CE): During the so called Tantric Renaissance of the middle ages there was a revival of Tantra in Kashmir, Bengal and South India, producing numerous teachers and texts, most notably Abhinava Gupta, author of the encyclopedic text Tantraloka. During this period, many other texts on Tantra were written, often in the style of conversations between Shiva and his wife Parvati, including Vijnana Bhairava Tantra, Kularnava Tantra, Shiva Samhita, Hatha Yoga Pradipika

and many others. Based on these texts, most Western scholars date
the beginning of Tantra history to this period, but many Indian
scholars and gurus, such as Anandamurtii, date Tantra to a much
earlier period. Some scholars trace the origin of Hatha Yoga to
Adi Shakanra (800 AD), who was believed to be an incarnation
of Shiva, others to Matsyendranatha (1000 AD) and his Natha
sect of Tantric yogis. It is said that Matsyendranatha received his
teachings from Shiva, thus linking his instructions to the tradition
of the much older lineage of Shaiva Tantra.

Lakulisha (50 BCE): At the beginning of our era, a clandestine
group of yogis led by Lakulisha re-awaken the old Shaiva tradition,
or Tantra, during a time when both the Vedic culture and Buddhism was in decline. According to the Puranas as well as his own
disciples, Lakulisha (the Club-bearing Lord) is considered to be the
twenty-eight manifestation of Shiva. In the Kurma Purana (chapter
53) it is predicted that a great, wandering yogi, or Maheshvara,
(another name for Shiva) would be reborn as Lakulin or Nakulisha
who would re-establish the ancient way of the Pashupata tradition,
the original Tantra tradition of Shiva. Lakulisha himself belonged
to the Kalamukha (Black Face) sect. It is said that he restored the
practices of Hatha Yoga, Tantrism and the cosmological ideas of
Samkhya (Danielou, 1987).

Patanjali's Yoga Sutras (200 BCE): This text, sometimes
termed Classical Yoga, is also considered by some scholars, such
as Georg Feuerstein, to be the beginning of yoga history, since it
is the first time the main ethical and spiritual practices of yoga are
combined in one system termed Asthtanga Yoga, or Raja Yoga.
Some scholars and schools of yoga characterize Patanjali's system
as Kriya Yoga (Feuerstein, 1998) and also to have originated in
Tantra (Anandamurtii, 1982) thus indicating the intimate link
between all yoga practice and Tantra. Other scholars remind us
that Patanjali's system follows in the tradition of Samkhya Yoga,
India's oldest philosophy; also termed Kapilasya Tantra, from its
founder Kapila (the one with brown skin). The earliest textual

evidence of Samkhya emerged around 700 BCE (Danielou, 1987), but Ananadmurtii claims that Kapila lived around 1500 BCE, at the time of Krishna, the Godman in the Bhagavad Gita, and that the system of Asthanga Yoga originated with Shiva, thousands of years before Patanjali. Furthermore, Anandamurtii also contends that the eight limbs of yoga—yama and niyama (ethics), asana (posture practice), pranayama (breath control), pratyahara (sense withdrawal), dharana (concentration), dhyana (meditation), samadhi (spiritual union)—is the heart of Tantric practice and originated with Shiva.

Gosala (500 BCE): During this period, Buddhism and Jainism was on the rise and Vedic society was beginning to decline. This was also the time of the Sramana movement, a yogic culture independent of Vedic hegemony. The roots of this culture lies in the ancient Shaiva tradition. Many centuries later, these two great cultural rivers of Indian antiquity, which had merged over thousands of years of migration, warfare and cultural co-mingling, became known as the Hindu tradition (about 1000 AD). It was during this pivotal time in history, shortly before the arrival of the historical Buddha, that Gosala emerged as a Shaiva Tantric revivalist among various groups of yogis, such as the Ajivikas, the Kapalikas and the Kalamukhas. Gosala became the teacher of both the Buddha and Mahavira (the founder of the Jain religion) for several years, and he sought to reinstate the philosophical and rational aspects of the ancient Shaiva culture, which was antagonistic to the Vedic caste system, and was populist, ecstatic and mystical in nature (Basham, 1987). Although some Jain texts claim that Mahavira was the teacher of Gosala, it is highly unlikely.

Samkhya (1500 BCE): According to Anandamurtii, Maharishi Kapila developed Samkhya philosophy around 1500 BCE. Most scholars "venerated him as the first exponent of *darshana shastra* and called him *adividvan* [first scholar]. This erudite personality of Rarh [Western Bihar] enumerated the fundamental causes of the mystery of this creation and presented them in a systematic way before the society of scholars." (Anandamurtii, 1982) Recent scholarship and the finding of ancient manuscripts lend support to the claim that Samkhya represents a non-Vedic system of dualist philosophy which is Shaiva Tantric in nature (Danielou, 1989). Some scholars assert that Samkhya may be the oldest school of Indian philosophy and influenced major schools of yoga philosophy, as well as Buddhism and Jainism. These scholars place the earliest references to Samkhya ideas in the Vedic period literature of India from 1500 BCE, an indication of Vedic texts assimilating non-Vedic ideas. (Larson, Potter, Bhattacharya, 2014)

Yoga and the Vedas (2000 BCE and onwards): Yoga is a spiritual path, which many scholars believe originated in the four Vedas. There are signs of yogic and especially Tantric practice in some of these texts, most notably the Atharvaveda, but on the whole these practices did not originate in the Vedic culture. Instead, yoga emerged from Shaiva Tantra and was absorbed into Vedic and Brahmanical culture after the Vedic Aryans migrated to India and, through conflict and assimilation, mingled with the native culture. The wisdom of Tantra was later expressed by various teachers as different forms of refined philosophy in the so-called fifth Veda, in texts such as the Brahmanas, the Bhagavad Gita, and the Upanishads, which were written from around 800 BCE and onwards.

Non-Vedic Yoga (5000 BCE and onwards): New scholarship now assert that yoga originated outside the Vedas in the Sramana period (500 BCE) among a group of wandering ascetics called Ajivikas, or beggars. (Mallinson and Singleton, 2017). The Indian scholar A. L. Basham remind us, however, that the term Ajivka "applied to the whole of the non-Aryan population" (Basham, 1981), thus indicating, as does other scholars, that yoga certainly had non-Vedic roots, and came from Shaiva Tantric "beggars" with cultural roots much older than 500 BCE. As Anandamurtii and Danielou asserts, yoga emerged from the ancient soil of the Shaiva culture of India, perhaps as early as 5000 BCE.

Tantric Yoga (5000 BCE and onwards): A group of scholars, practitioners and gurus claim that "the ascetics" who invented yoga, the Shaiva Tantrics, are the main source of not only yoga but also Ayurvedic medicine, the musical scale, and alchemy. According to some interpretations of archeology, passages in the Puranas, and the writings of, among others, Alain Danielou, Prasad Lalan Singh, N.N. Bhattacaryya, R. P. Chanda, and Shrii Shrii Anandamurtii, this important culture, which is still very much alive in India, and which over time was absorbed into Vedic culture, originated with Shiva (Anandamurtii, 1993), who is well known in India as The King of Yoga. This yogic or Tantric culture, whose goals are primarily to seek spiritual enlightenment, is very diverse and rich and in many ways quite different from the "health and feel-good" posture yoga movement in the contemporary Western world.

The short narrative above, spanning over five millennia of Indian history, depict the long, complex and illustrious history of yoga. In this book, we will look at all of these possible ways to view the origins and developments of yoga, but mainly focus on the last and longest historical timeline, as it naturally includes all of the other timelines. We will investigate the entire span of Indian history and thus the history of one of the world's oldest spiritual ways of life from the perspective of its early roots—the tradition of Shaiva Tantra.

Chapter One
Yoga, Tantra and the Vedas

IT HAS BEEN COMMONLY accepted that yoga originated in the Vedas, India's oldest sacred texts. "In its oldest known form," writes prolific yoga scholar Georg Feuerstein, "yoga appears to have been the practice of disciplined introspection, or meditative focusing, in conjunction with sacrificial rituals." The rituals Feuerstein refer to are those found in the four Vedas, the ancient Sanskrit texts of the Vedic priests. These Brahmin priests sacrificed animals or used ghee and milk in elaborate prayer rituals as offerings to the Gods in heaven. They poured ghee into fire pits in the hope of a rich harvest, good health, more children or victory in battle.

Yoga, according to Feuerstein, originated in the Vedic Yoga Period about 3-4000 BCE, flourished further in the Epic Yoga Period of the Mahabharata and the Upanishads around 800-500 BCE, culminated in the Classical Yoga Period with the writing of the Yoga Sutras of Patanjali around 200 BCE, and then peaked during the Tantra Renaissance Period from 500 CE to about 1500 CE.

Since the Classical Yoga Period of Patanjali's Yoga Sutras onwards, there is little disagreement among scholars today about the development of yoga. The main disagreements about yoga history relates to the early roots of yoga: did yoga originate in the Vedas or outside the Vedas; did yoga originate in the Sramana movement or much earlier—in the Tantric Shaiva culture of prehistoric India? These are some of the main questions addressed in this book.

Modern Hatha Yoga

Modern Hatha Yoga, or posture yoga, with its emphasis on physical exercises and less on meditation, is no more than 100 years old. As mentioned above, this type of yoga originated in the 1920s with Krishnamacarya in Mysore, India. In the 1960s and 1970s, his well-known students, B.K. S. Iyengar, Patthabi Jois and A.K. Deshikachar brought new and refined versions of his teachings to the West. The Western students of these teachers departed even further from tradition by inventing yet newer versions of posture yoga—a popular pastime which continue to spread in yoga studios, fitness centers, and in social media today.

Guru Yoga and Tantra Yoga

Although yoga in the popular media today is largely synonymous with its physical postures, it is also a spiritual path of study, meditation, prayer and chanting. A Vedantic version of this latter form of yoga migrated from India to the West with Swami Vivekananda, a charismatic orator from Kolkata, Bengal. Vivekananda emphasized the importance of meditation and yoga philosophy when he arrived in the US in 1893 to give a riveting and memorable speech at the Parliament of the World's Religions in Chicago. He promoted Vedantic philosophy and Raja Yoga— another name for Patanjali's Classical Yoga. To him yoga was a spiritual science more than a religion and certainly not just an exercise regimen. In fact, Vivekananda de-emphasized the yoga postures so popular with Westerners today.

In the 1920s, another Bengali, the handsome Swami Yogananda reached the shores of America wearing long, dark hair and a striking orange turban. After having a vision in his meditation that he should sail to the West, he asked his guru, Shrii Yukteshvar for permission to travel to America. Like his predecessor Vivekananda, Yogananda also promoted meditation, but he combined it with yoga postures through a system he called Kriya Yoga, yet another term used in Patanjali's Yoga Sutras. Yogananda received a warm welcome in America and soon founded the organization Self-Realization Fellowship to promote his teachings. His book, *Autobiography of a Yogi*, published in 1946, is considered a modern, spiritual classic and is promoted by his organization with the slogan "The Book that Changed the Lives of Millions." In keeping with the tradition of his Guru, Shrii Yuktesvar, Yogananda taught a system combining Raja Yoga (meditation) and Hatha Yoga (postures). This tradition goes back to the Tantric Hatha Yogis of the Middle Ages who always emphasized that Hatha Yoga without Raja Yoga was "useless."

In the footsteps of these holy men came other traditional yogis, some of which taught a system of yoga they termed Tantra. Swami Muktananda, a teacher of Kashmir Shaiva Tantra, introduced *shaktipat*, a form of initiation in which a guru awakens in the disciple the primal force of *kundalini*, or Shakti. His organization, Siddha Yoga, continues to thrive today and has produced several prominent scholars of Tantra, most notably Christopher Wallis, a popular author and teacher. Many other swamis and gurus, including Swami Satchitanananda and Swami Vishnudevananda, introduced a form of yoga in the West in which both yoga and meditation, both Raja Yoga and Hatha Yoga are practiced together. Some teachers and schools of yoga, such as the Indian Bihar School of Yoga, which has many centers in the West calls this combination of yoga simply Tantra Yoga. It is this form of yoga, they claim, which is the origin of all forms of yoga.

India produced another prominent, modern teacher, also from Bengal, and who likewise promoted yoga as Tantra, namely Shrii Shrii Anandamurti, a renaissance man with impressive linguistic skills, extraordinary powers of the mind, and a prolific author. He wrote hundreds of books on topics from farming to economics, from art to Tantra, and he composed over 5000 songs. He was also a Tantric guru who, in no uncertain terms, claimed that "it would be incorrect to regard Tantra as a recent version of those Vedic rituals." According to him, Tantra represent the ancient culture of India, and even today "the civilization of India is intrinsically Tantric." To him, Tantra is also the ancient source of yoga. But unlike the popular idea that Tantra is a sexual practice, he emphasized that it is "a way of life" which includes yoga and meditation as its core lifestyle practices. Yoga, according to Ananadamurtii, represents the subtler aspects and the goal of Tantra. Drawing on old, textual sources, he explained that yoga, according to Tantra, literally means *union* and the word's inner, spiritual meaning is the transcendental union between the human mind and the cosmic mind, an enlightened experience which can occur during deep states of meditation (Anandamurtii, 1993).

Yoga and Its Non-Vedic Roots

If yoga did not originate in the Vedas 2500 years ago, when did it originate? In 2017, James Mallinson and Mark Singleton, two Oxford and Cambridge educated yogi scholars and practitioners, published the formidable book *Roots of Yoga*, in which they claim that yoga originated in the Sramana movement, perhaps as early as 1000 BCE and flourished as an ascetic and distinct school of yogis around 500 BCE. These wandering yogis were thus contemporary with Buddha, and they were neither Vedic priests nor did they engage in the ritualistic killing of animals during the Vedic rituals. Instead, they engaged in meditation, prayer and various physical exercises and penances, and, according to these two authors, it is from these groups of mendicants as well as from Buddhism and Jainism that yoga originated.

More specifically, these authors claim, yoga originated with a small group of ascetics called Ajivikas, wandering mendicants who did not adhere to the norms of caste and rituals of Vedic society. Tantra author Prasad Lalan Singh reminds us, however, that the Ajivikas were actually Tantric yogis, and N. N. Bhattacaryya, author of *The History of the Tantric Religion* writes that an Ajivika also signified "the other," all those outside the Vedic society, not just a specific sect of yogis. To respected Orientalist and historian Alain Danielou, "these others" were all those not following the Vedic tradition, the followers of Shiva. "The Vedas, the texts of the Aryan invaders," he writes, "fulminate against the worshippers of the phallus and the forms of the Shaivite cult." In other words, in order to understand the history of yoga and its origins in Tantra, we need to understand the history of India and the often contentious conflicts between the Vedic Aryans and the Tantric Dravidians, Mongolians and Austrics, all the indigenous peoples who inhabited India before the Aryan migration.

The Vedic Aryan migration, the conflict between the Vedic Aryans and their Brahmin priests and the Shaiva Tantrics, is often either a very contentious issue or completely glossed over in writings about Indian history. Most yoga scholars do not even mention it, and if they do, they often claim, against all evidence, that the Vedic Aryans were indigenous to India and represent all that is great about yoga and Indian culture. In order to understand the history of yoga, we must therefore understand the perennial conflict between the incoming Vedic Aryans and the indigenous Shaiva Tantrics. This conflict is partly based on race (the Aryans were Caucasian), partly based on religion (the Vedic Aryans were ritualists and believed in the caste system, while the Shaiva Tantrics were meditating yogis), and partly based on class (the Vedic Aryans became the dominating class while the Shaiva peoples most often came from the underclass and the casteless). In nearly all the writings on yoga history by Western scholars these important issues are hardly ever mentioned.

As noted by Bhattacharyya, most yoga scholars have missed to describe the common attitude among the upper castes in India that "whatever is noble and praiseworthy in Hinduism is found in this so called Aryan tradition, i.e. the Vedic texts and Brahmanical literature, and all the barbarous and degraded aspects attributed to Tantra are derived from the uncivilized non-Aryans." It is this bias toward the greatness of everything Vedic which has colored much of the writings on yoga history so far. Moreover, according to Danielou, the Shaivite Samkhya philosophy "of which yoga is the experimental method" is also the original source of yogic, Ayurvedic and Tantric philosophy. And if Anandamurtii is correct in saying that Maharishi Kapila, the sage who developed Samkhya philosophy, lived as a contemporary of Krishna, around 1500 BCE, then non-Vedic yoga is at least 1000 years older than proposed by Singleton and Mallinson, and nearly 2500 years older than that proposed by science writer William Broad, who stated in an interview that "yoga originated in a Tantric sex cult in the middle ages." (NPR, 2012) As noted above, yoga is not only much older in its homeland India than previously thought, yoga also migrated West long before Vivekananda came to America in 1883. The Danish Gundesrup cauldron (500 BCE), is a silver bowl depicting a yogi-like figure surrounded by animals and strikingly similar to the Pashupatinat figure from 2500 BCE in India. This, and other archeological signs, such as yogi-like stone statues found in France, stone carvings of yoga postures in Sweden, and a Viking yogi in Norway, points toward a migration of yoga culture into Europe as early as several thousand years ago—at least symbolic and mythological expressions of this ancient, esoteric culture. (Armstrong Oma, 2008)

Chapter Two
The Union of Tantra and Yoga

IN A YOGA JOURNAL article in 2007 by Nora Isaacs it was predicted that Tantra would be the "next evolution" in Western yoga. With the popularity of books such as the *Radiance Sutras* by Lorin Roche and the proliferation of workshops, writings, podcasts and videos by Tantric scholars Douglas Brooks, Sally Kempton, Christopher Wallis, and many others, Tantric philosophy, yoga, and meditation practices are having increased influence in Western yoga circles today.

Most of the yoga students I encounter in my workshops, however, know very little about Tantra. Many mistakenly think it is an esoteric sexual practice, and only a few are aware of Tantra's long and deep relationship to yoga, even fewer know that it may in fact be the origin of all of yoga's numerous posture and meditation practices. So, let us take a closer look at what Tantra is, where it originated, and how relevant this ancient wisdom tradition is for modern yogis.

The Indus Valley: The Roots of Tantra and Yoga

About 4500 years ago, an unknown artist in the Indus Valley created an enigmatic figure with an animal head sitting in a yogi-like posture. Esteemed art historian Thomas McEvilley wrote in his extensive essay, *An Archeology of Yoga*, that this seal, of which there are at least four different versions, depicts a Tantric yogi practicing the *goraksha-asana* posture. The purpose of sitting in the goraksha-asana posture, according to various tantric texts, is to transform the sexual energy into kundalini, or spiritual energy.

To McEvilley, Marshall, and many Indian researchers, this historically important seal is a symbolic representation of the Dravidian yoga culture of the Indus Valley. This sophisticated, urban culture, where yogic practice had already developed, was allegedly destroyed by invading Vedic Aryans around 2000 BCE. As noted earlier, recent research, however, combining genetics with archeology and linguistics, as well as the chronicles of the Puranas and the oral teachings of Tantric teachers, has shifted the timeline of the Vedic Aryan migration into India further back, to at least 5000 BCE. It is also now believed that the Indus Valley civilization was destroyed by climate change—dry, hot weather and lack of water—rather than a violent invasion.

While the Dravidian Tantric culture had evolved from a shamanistic society were phallus and mother worship was common, the central focus of the Aryan religion was the sacrificial fire rituals of the priests, where prayers to the Gods and Goddesses in heaven were crafted, first to appease their wrath, then to request their boons and graces. The Vedic Aryans were cattle herders and warriors, according to N. N. Bhattacharyya, an historian and author of several books on the history of Tantra. They came to India, he writes, much like the British "with a 'civilizing mission' to bear the 'white man's burden.'" During these prehistoric times, the "aboriginal Indians were 'civilized' by the Aryans who came from outside." According to the Vedic Aryans themselves, Bhattacharya notes, "whatever is noble and praiseworthy in Hindusim is found in [the] so called Aryan tradition, i.e. the Vedic texts and the Brahmanical literature, and all the barbarous and degraded aspects attributed to tantra are derived from the uncivilized non-Aryans. This idea was also shared by the learned Indians who belonged mostly, if not exclusively, to the upper strata of society and took pride in thinking of themselves as direct descendants of the great Aryan race." Consequently, there has been a bias toward the Vedic and Brahmanical as the source of yoga and Tantra since ancient times.

"The Aryans were not the original inhabitants of the present India," writes the Tantric guru Anandamurtii, whose essays are today regularly printed in major Indian newspapers. The white complexioned Aryans "contemptuously called the much darker indigenous population whom they defeated in battle, Anaryas," [non-Aryans]. Anandamurtii writes in the same essay that the original inhabitants of India at that time were often labeled as asuras (monsters), raksasas (demons), and pashus, (beasts), thus emphasizing, and soon institutionalizing, a racial and social divide that he says has plagued India ever since. The Vedic Aryans, who first settled in Kash (later called Kashmeru, or Kashmira, and today Kahsmir) "did not give up their Vedic studies," he writes, but in the field of spirituality "they did cultivate the indigenous Indian Tantra." It is for this reason, according to Anandamurtii, that some of the earliest Vedic texts, especially the Atharvaveda, were strongly influenced by Tantric thought. "In the subtle philosophy of the Atharvaveda, particularly the *Nirsimha Tapaniya Shruti*, there is a far greater influence of the non-Aryan Tantra than of the Aryan Veda." (Anandamurtii, 1993)

Veda and Tantra: Cultural Clash and Integration

According to Dr. Spencer Wells—writer of the PBS/National Geographic documentary *Journey of Man*, and a landmark population geneticist—the first wave of modern humans migrated from Africa into India about 50,000 years ago, some settled in South India, the rest moved onwards to Australia. The second wave arrived about 25,000 years ago. They became known as the Dravidians. The first members of the third major wave arrived between 7-5000 BCE; these became known as the Vedic Aryans, and they carried the so called M17 genetic marker. The Vedic Aryans original homeland was Southern Russia and the Ukraine. From there, they moved East in search of a better homeland for their large cattle and sheep herds. In India today, "around 35 percent of the men in Hindi-speaking populations carry the M17 marker," writes Dr. Wells in his book *Deep Ancestry*, "whereas the frequency in the neighboring communities of Dravidian speakers is only about 10 percent." Other genetic studies point out that men from higher castes, such as Vedic Brahmins, have a higher concentration of these "white genes." (Wells, 2003)

During the peak of the Indus Valley civilization, around 2500 BCE, when the yogic seal of the Pashupatinat figure was artfully constructed, there were two major religions or wisdom traditions in India, both of whom had their origins several thousand years earlier. Namely the Aryan Vedic religion and the Dravidian Tantric religion, also called the Shaiva religion, since its followers attributed their ancient teachings to Shiva. "Shaivism," writes Alain Danielou, a distinguished Indologist and author of many books on Indian philosophy and history, "was always the religion of the people." This religion, he writes, was "preserved by communities of wandering ascetics living on the fringe of official [Aryan controlled] society, whom the Aryans scornfully called Yati (wanderer), Vratya (untouchable), or Ajivika (beggar)." Since the dawn of Indian civilization, then, there has been both a gradual blending and a clash between the Vedic and the Shiva-oriented civilizations, between the priestly religion of ritualism and belief and the yogic religion of meditation and Tantric practice, between the upper caste Brahmins and the lower castes. For this reason, many scholars, and most definitely most Tantric teachers and scholars, distinguish between the Vedic and the Tantric aspects of Hinduism. (Danielou, 2006)

Yoga Journal, the most popular yoga magazine in the world, also promotes the view that yoga originated in the Vedas. The main proponents of this chronology in the West are the prolific writers Georg Feuerstein and David Frawley, who claim there was never an Aryan migration into India. The most vocal adherents to this view, however, belong to the followers of the Hindutva movement, who continue to believe in the superiority of the Vedic religion, claiming—against linguistic, genetic and archeological evidence—there was never an Aryan migration into India. (Frawley, 1996) To the Hindutvas, the Pauspatinath figure is "proof" of the Vedic origin of yoga. To them, the proponents of the Aryan migration theory into India are "racist" and "Euro-centric." Ironically, the so called Euro-centric scholars and writers, including myself, are in fact claiming that the greatest contributors to yoga are not the white Aryan invaders but rather the indigenous Dravidians.

The Hindu nationalists dismiss any link between the Pashupatinat figure and the culture from which it was crafted, the Shaiva tradition of the Dravidians and their contribution to Indian society in general and to yoga and Tantra in particular. Therefore, "Tantra and the Veda are two different currents of India's cultural life," writes Tantra scholar Lalan Prasad Singh, who distinguishes between Tantra as the essence of yogic practice and the Vedas as a religious and philosophical "school of thought." But both systems are complimentary, he writes, and both have been pivotal in the evolution of the cultural and spiritual life of India. (Singh, 1972)

In *The Roots of Yoga*, Mallinson and Singleton, downplay the importance of the Pashupatinat seal and its Tantric origins, while also arguing it is entirely speculative to claim that "the Vedic corpus provide any evidence of systematic yoga practice" (Mallinson and Singleton, 2017)

As noted before, I disagree with the first argument, and I only partially agree with the second. This does not mean that there are no traces of yoga or Tantra practice at all in the early Vedic texts. Since these texts were Vedic, not Tantric, the mention of such practices, such as in the Atharvaveda, including the practice of "visionary meditation," pranayama and a long Rigvedic hymn to a "long-haired sage" (most likely the dreadlocked Shiva), only underscores the significant influence Shaiva Tantra had on these texts in particular and the Vedic Aryan peoples in general, even at such an early stage in history. More importantly, the lack of textual evidence is also due to the Tantric guru-tradition itself, which was, and still is, largely a secret and oral tradition. The teachings were transmitted and remembered in the form of sutras (metaphoric and philosophical chants), mantras (incantations) and yantras (symbols) for thousands of years and would therefore not have been written down in these early texts. It was only thousands of years later, when a written alphabet had been developed, that some of the early Tantric teachings began to be widely incorporated not only into the Vedic texts, but also many other Hindu religious scriptures.

The ancient Indians, including the Vedic Aryans, developed techniques to memorize and impart their knowledge, while maintaining exceptional accuracy for thousands of years before and after the texts were written down. Many of the ancient Shaiva Tantric teachings were contained in texts called the Agamas and Nigamas, as well as in the Puranas (ancient chronicles). Thousands of yogic texts still exist which have never before been translated into English., most of them Tantric in nature. The most secret initiation and meditation techniques, however, were never recorded in the texts; they were passed on verbally, sometimes only in whispers, from teacher to student. Many of the Tantric teachings were also incorporated in texts that we do not consider Tantric and only an expert guru or scholar would be able to distinguish its unique character. Anandamurtii, for example, presented many discourses based entirely on Tantric teachings scattered throughout these texts. (Anandamurtii, 1993)

According to Alain Danielou, the influence of the ancient Shaiva Tantra has been so significant in India that «the Hindu religion, as it is practiced today, is Tantric in character, based almost exclusively on the Agamas.» Large parts of the Bhagavad Gita, for example, is, according to M.R. Sakhare's *History and Philosophy of the Lingayat Religion*, based on the Parameshvara Agama, while the Shvetashvatara Upanishad, which has been added to the Yajurveda, is also based on the Agamas, and is a foundational text of Tantric

Shaivism. (Sakhare, 1978). As we can see, the Vedic and the Tantric traditions of India have run both paralell and in comingled streams since the early dawn of Indian history. But it is the Shaiva Tantric tradition, not the Vedic tradition, which contain the main roots to the large and ancient tree of Tantra—from which the many later branches of yoga have sprung.

Scattered throughout the most important Vedic, Upanishadic and Brahmanical texts, we will find the wisdom teachings of Tantra since the dawn of Indian civilization. Mostly these teachings are categorized as yoga, but as many scholars and indigenous teachers maintain, we might as well call them Tantra, because the source, philosophy and practice of Tantra and yoga are broadly the same. That said, there are of course many distinct philosophical schools of yoga and Tantra, but Shaiva Tantra is the main source of yoga, both in the form of hatha yoga, or posture practices, as well as Raja Yoga. Thus, even the Yoga Sutras of Patanjali, which few scholars recognize as Tantric, are, from this perespective, Tantric to the core. For as it is said in the Shiva Samhita, an important Tantric text of the middle ages, without Raja Yoga, the practice of Hatha Yoga is «useless».

Yoga scholars James Mollinson and Mark Singleton favor the view that yoga developed long after the four Vedas were composed, around 1000 BCE onwards. Yoga, these scholars claim, grew out of Buddhist, Jain and Ajivaka ascetic practices and the philosophy of yoga was outlined in the Brahmanas, the Upanishads and the Bhagvad Gita. As we have seen above, there is a third view, not as common perhaps, but which, to me, is more plausible: that yoga in the from of Tantra is an ancient and paralell tradition to the Vedic, and that it originated with the Shaiva tradition of the ancient Dravidians. This ancient tradition, with its hatha yoga, meditation and breathing practices, even its medicinal tradition (for it is said in many texts and by many traditional teachers that Shiva is the father of not only yoga but also Ayurveda), deeply influenced and flavored all of the great yogic texts that followed in its wake: the Agamas, the Upanishads, the Bhagavad Gita, the Samkhya, the Yoga Sutras, and of course the Tantras of the middle ages. (Mallinson and Singleton, 2017)

In summary, there are four main reasons the history of yoga and Tantra needs to be revised so that the important role Shaiva Tantra has played in shaping the history and practice of yoga can be appreciated: 1) Most of yoga and Tantra history has been written by the dominant classes, those whose caste, social, and intellectual loyalties can be traced back through history to the Vedic warriors who have dominated the political, economic and socail life of India from ancient times until today; 2) the Western academic methods of dating and cataloging information has paid little attention to the fact that yoga and Tantra are largely oral traditions that are often thousands of years older than the written texts of the same traditions; 3) few Indian or Western scholars have themselves practiced the various lineages they have been studying, thus many facts, timelines, and teachings pertaining to the various lineages and their founders have not been noted; 4) there is often a Western bias toward searching for «the truth» and the «correct history» in published texts without complementing the textual study with the study of the oral teachings and the living traditions themselves and its authorized teachers and practicing scholars.

Many students of yoga, especially those undergoing yoga teacher training, are introduced to the Yoga Sutras of Patanjali. It is commonly accepted by scholars and practitioners alike that this text represent the culmination of the ancient yoga tradition's spiritual quest. These so-called Classical Yoga teachings, most scholars believe, are the confluence of a long and complex development that emerged from yoga's archaic beginnings in the Vedas about 2000 years before Patanjali wrote the Yoga Sutras.

Adopted by Yoga Journal and most Western yogis as the "official" starting point of yoga, the idea that yoga originated with the Vedic tradition has been promoted by the prolific writings of yoga scholars such as Georg Feuerstein and David Frawley as well as by many religious university scholars around the world. The current Indian government, headed by Prime Minister Modi, is also favoring this view. The most aggressive proponents of this version of Indian history, however, is the Hindutva movement. Their controversial views, sometimes also associated with both anti-Muslim and anti-European sentiments, stem from the idea that Hindutva, or Hinduness, or Vedic culture, represents the true culture of India. Despite genetic, linguistic and archeological evidence to the contrary, the Hindutva also believe that the Vedic Aryans are indigenous to India. Interestingly, Feuerstein and Frawley's path-breaking book, *In Search of the Cradle of Human Civilization*, which attempts to prove there was never a Vedic Aryan invasion or migration into India, thus attempting to overturn prevailing academic opinions about Indian history, was funded by the Hindutva movement. (Frawley, 1996)

For the Hindutva, the idea that the Aryans came from outside India, represent European appropriation and outright racism, a false idea rooted in the superiority of white culture and race. To them, the Aryan and Vedic culture is not only indigenous to India, it also represent all that is great about India, especially the wisdom of Vedic religious ideas and its many offshoots, including yoga. Because, according to them there is no evidence of an invasion destroying the Indus Valley civilization at that time; since the Indus Valley was most likely destroyed by climate change, not war.

Discussing the history of India and the roots of yoga, a practice people in the West associate with promoting health, tranquility, and spirituality, is therefore sometimes a contentious affair. Contrary ideas about the origins of yoga brings up heated arguments in chat rooms, on blogs and on Facebook, between scholars and practitioners, between Indians and Westerners, between modern posture yogis and more traditional yogis. The interconnection between Tantra and yoga is one of the reasons behind the contentions. Another reason is the philosophical and practical polarity between theoretical scholarship and practitioners of the tradition.

A third is the often dynamic contention between scholar practitioners and experienced practitioners who are not academic scholars but nevertheless are deeply schooled in the practice and philosophy of their tradition.

As a non-academic scholar and practitioner who has learned from within the tradition through the teachings of a Tantric guru, I find myself in the interesting position of practicing a form of contemplative yoga that Patanjali outlined in the Yoga Sutras. A practice, which for me, is also called Tantra. In today's yoga teacher trainings in the West, however, most students are given a superficial introduction to Patanjali's yoga philosophy, while the meditative teachings and practices that the Yoga Sutras represent are rarely taught or practiced at all. There are simply very few qualified teachers who has the practical knowledge to impart these more esoteric teachings. Thus, Western yoga is still primarily a fitness practice with a focus on the third limb of Patanjali's teachings, namely the postures.

But the Yoga Sutras is not a manual on Hatha Yoga. The book mentions only four different asana positions for meditation and emphasizes their importance as "comfortable seats" in order to sustain deep and long meditation. There is textual evidence of the practice of such postures in India since at least 1000 BCE and, as mentioned earlier, archeological evidence since at least 2500 BCE in the form of the Pashupatinath seal. The textual evidence of the term hatha yoga, however, did not occur before the 11th century CE with the advent of the Tantric Nath yogis, such as the famous Goraksanath.

The meditational pranayama practice described in the Yoga Sutras, a form of which I practice, is not the same as the Hatha Yoga pranayama practice, such as the breath of fire, used by many hatha yogis in yoga studios all over the world today. In my Tantric tradition, there is a clear distinction between hatha yoga practices (such as asana and pranayama) and the more mental or spiritual practices (of Raja Yoga), or pranayama seated in siddhasana pose using a mantra and focusing on specific chakras. In other words, there is often a difference between what is taught, or alluded to, in the texts and what is taught orally from guru to disciple through the process of initiation. Therefore, the Yoga Sutras is mainly a philosophical text, while the practical teachings are taught through the process of various initiation sessions, during which the teachings are hardly ever written down but rather passed on orally until the student remembers how to perform the subtle lessons of the practice. In other words, there is a difference between Hatha Yoga and Raja Yoga, and in the traditional form of Tantra, these practices are complimentary.

Therefore, the most essential practices of Tantra and yoga—such as meditation practices during which specific mantras most suited to a particular individual are taught—are not found in texts nor in the vast selection of more commonly known mantras. Rather, the texts are at best complimentary teachings, or signposts hinting at the inner meaning of the practical meditations, which are only revealed through one's own practical experiences and only to a lesser degree through academic study. Indeed, without that practical background, the academic scholar will miss out on quite a lot of the tradition's inner wisdom teachings. Similarly, the average yoga student in the West today have not been exposed to most of the oral teachings that have been the core lessons of these traditions for many millennia.

What is Tantra?

The Sanskrit word Tantra has many meanings. Etymologically, Tantric scholar Christopher Wallis writes that the Sanskrit root word *tan* means to propagate, expand on, liberate, and that *tra* means to save or protect. Indian Sanskrit scholar and Tantric guru Ananadamurtii breaks up the root words differently and gives them a slightly altered meaning. His interpretation of *tra* is to liberate us from *ta*, from limitations, from bondage. Tantra, then, can be described as a path of liberation and expansion from bondage.

The word Tantra is also used to describe a system, practice, or science. India's earliest philosophy, Samkhya, is therefore often referred to as Kapilasya Tantra—the system of Kapila, named after the man who developed the Samkhya philosophy. Similarly, even aspects of Patanjali's Yoga Sutras, are sometimes also referred to as Kriya and Tantra, and in Ayurveda, many of the various healing systems are also termed Tantra.

So, if we strip away the various philosophies of yoga and look at what yoga is in practical terms, then what emerges at the core is Tantra as a practical system of religion or spirituality, a system of physical and mental transformation, a practice promoting healing and liberation of the human body and mind. In the book a *History of the Tantric Religion,* N. N. Bhattacharyya writes that Tantra grew out of early shamanism, a system which developed from the early worship of the *linga* and *yoni* to the metaphysical concepts of Purusha and Prakrti in Samkhya, or Shiva and Shakti in Tantra, representing the polarities of nature, the male and female principles of creation. The practice of yoga, in which the human body was "the abode of all the mysteries of the universe" emerged from these worshippers of the duality of creation. This non-Vedic system, where some groups worshipped Shakti and others Shiva, Bhattacharyya points out, represent the origins of yoga. (Bhattacharyya, 1999)

Bhattacharyya also points out the deep rift between early Vedic and Tantric cultures, which stems from the religious and racial clash of peoples, between the invading Vedic Aryans and the indigenous peoples of India. He also points out that many Vedic Brahmins, even though they over time would take up yoga, could "not give up their Brahminical prejudices despite their conversion to Tantrism." They instead attempted "to demonstrate the Vedic origin of Tantra, and so they often twisted Vedic passages to suit their own purpose." Such attempts also influenced the first modern writers of yoga and Tantra, including Sir John Woodroffe, Gopinath Kaviraj, and most of the contemporary writers on yoga have followed suit, to wrongly attribute the origin of yoga and Tantra to the Vedas. (Bhattacharyya, 1999)

The Importance of Tantra in Yoga History

Some contemporary Western scholars, including Georg Feuerstein, are also reminding us that Tantra played an important role in shaping the origins of yoga as we know it today. Contemporary Tantric teacher Anandamurtii claimed that the roots of the controversy over ancient Indian history, and thus the roots of yoga, lies at the heart of the ancient conflict between the Vedic Aryans and the Shaiva culture of the Dravidians; a struggle, he reminds us, that is depicted in the famous epic battles in the Mahabharata and the stories of the Ramayana, a conflict which, in cultural, political, religious and economic terms, has continued into our times.

The clash of ideas in the yoga community today is largely a continuation of these two worldviews: one claiming yoga originated in the Vedic system and one believing it is of Tantric origin. In the scholarly community some claim, based on certain textual evidences, that Tantra is only 1500 years old and those scholars who, based on textual, genetic, archeological, linguistic and other evidences, claim the tradition stems from the much older Shaiva culture of India, which is perhaps as old as 6-7000 years.

Whether we think of yoga as only the practice of postures, or the whole plethora of yogic practices—from the ethical tenets of yama and niyama to meditation, from pranayama to chakra visualizations—Patanjali's Yoga Sutras, today hailed as the main text on yoga philosophy, contains a lot more Tantric wisdom than religious insights drawn from the ancient Vedas.

Tantra:
The People's Religion and the Parallel Tradition

As in most other places where religion and the power of empires were linked, the Vedic hegemony was based on a schism of class, caste and socio-economic status. Historian N. N. Bhattacaryya says of this phenomenon that "the Vedas came to be looked upon as a symbol of spiritual knowledge, a very sacred and unchallengeable tradition… and a strong taboo for the ordinary people. It reached to the extent that if a Sudra [low caste] ventured to go through the Vedas to acquire knowledge of his own profession he was liable to receive punishment." He further states that what "was denied in the Vedic tradition, was naturally filled by the Tantras, which appeared as a parallel tradition."

Most importantly, perhaps, Bhattacharyya emphasizes that to understand the history of Tantra and thus yoga, we cannot solely rely on the "official" texts, which most Western scholars today proclaim as the main source of yogic practice and history. "In the quest for the foundation and early development of Tantrism," he writes, "we have to depend more on the parallel tradition itself as manifested in numerous non-Brahmanical and heterodox, scientific, and technological treatises, regional, tribal, proletarian and popular cults, beliefs, and practices and on the broad background of the history of Indian thought in general, rather than on surviving Tantric texts themselves which, valuable though they are in many respects, are in their present form burdened with superimposed elements and thus bear only a parochial and limited significance." (Bhattacharyya, 1999)

One more notable difference between the Vedic and the Tantric system, Bhattacharyya writes, is that in Tantra "external formalities in regard to the spiritual quest" was rejected. He also notes that many of the main teachers of the Tantric tradition, including the two most famous ones from the Natha sects in the Middle Ages,

Matsyendranatha and Goraksanatha, came "from the lower section of society." (Bhattacharyya, 1999)

One example of this cultural conflict between those who write the history of India from a Brahmanical and Vedic perspective, and those who write from a Tantric perspective can be seen in each perspective's understanding of the origin of Ayurveda. It is commonly understood by yoga students in the West that Ayurveda is a Vedic science, as that is how it has been taught in books written by David Frawley and others. Both Anandamurtii and Bhattacharyya, however, note that Ayurveda and medical alchemy in general has been an integral part of Tantra. "Indian medical sciences," writes Bhattachrayya, "as revealed in the Carakasamhita (the main text book of Ayurveda) is basically Tantric." He continues by pointing out that much of Western academic understanding of Tantra and Yoga is based on texts from the Common Era, while the Carakasamhita and other Tantric texts contains "information from the earlier Tantric tradition," from long before the Christian Era. In fact, at one point this important Ayurvedic text was also called Agnivesa Tantra. Anandamurtii suggests that the roots of Tantra goes even further back into human prehistory and claims that both Yoga and Ayurveda hail from the Tantric teachings of Shiva, the King of Yoga himself. (Bhattacharyya, 1999)

Tantra:
A Bridge Between Hatha Yoga and Raja Yoga

Most yoga scholars draw a distinct separation between Patanjali's Yoga Sutras and the teachings of the Tantric texts, basically claiming that Patanjali's Asthanga Yoga and Tantra are entirely different schools of yoga. But not everyone draws such a distinct separation between the two systems, especially not the indigenous teachers of the tradition.

When I learned Tantric meditation practices in India in the early 80s, I was taught techniques that are central to Patanjali's work. In his Yoga Sutras, the goal of yoga practice is inner peace, or, as he put it, "the cessation of the fluctuations of mental propensities." To reach this goal of spiritual tranquility, also termed Samadhi, he described the eight limbed path of Asthanga Yoga.

Ashtanga yoga was exactly what I was taught in the name of Tantra in India and Nepal. I was also told that Samadhi is the goal of Tantric meditation. Through oral transmission from my teachers, I was given detailed practices that are only philosophically or symbolically explained in the Yoga Sutras. Perhaps because so many scholars do not have practical experience with the traditions behind the texts and the philosophy, there is a tendency to separate Tantric practice from the philosophy of yoga. But as it is often said in Tantra circles: yoga is 99% practice and 1% theory.

According to teachers and writers such as Shrii Shrii Ananadamurtii, Alain Danielou and Lalan Prasad Singh, this system emerged from the ancient Tantric Shaiva tradition, and philosophically from Samkhya, the main religious and philosophical traditions of yoga in ancient India. It is also popularly believed in India that the techniques behind the eightfold path, and especially the Tantric teachings of mantra, kundalini and chakras, originated in antiquity with the legendary Shiva, the King of Yoga and the original teacher of Tantra. Many indigenous teachers of Ayurveda in Nepal and India will therefore address Shiva as the Father of Ayurveda. (Crow, 1997)

In the book *Laya Yoga* by Shyam Sundar Goswami, which Georg Feuerstein hails as "the last word on the chakras and the kundalini," Goswami explains that both Vedic and Tantric yoga has eight stages, the same eight limbs outlined in the form of Asthanga Yoga in Patanjali's Yoga Sutras. Goswami further explains that there are four main forms of Tantric yoga practice: Laya Yoga, Mantra Yoga, Hatha Yoga and Raja Yoga. (Goswami, 1999)

Therefore, the distinct lines many yoga scholars and practitioners today draw between the various forms of yoga and Tantra are artificial. Because, at their very roots, Tantra and yoga are intertwined, even synonymous paths that has meandered through time, eventually forming one single trunk. A large trunk we today simply call yoga. But it would be equally accurate to name the same trunk Tantra.

Not surprisingly, when Yogananda came to the shores of the United States in the 1920s, he taught yoga as a combination of Hatha Yoga and Raja Yoga, a style which he, like Patanjali, called Kriya Yoga. This eight-limbed style of yoga is what Anandamurtii and other yogi scholars in India sometimes refer to as Ashtanga Yoga and sometimes Tantra Yoga.

When B.K.S. Iyengar, Patthabi Jois, and T. K .V. Desikachar introduced yoga to the world a few decades after Yogananda, as students of Krishnamacarya, the father of modern posture yoga, however, their emphasis was mainly on the physical side of yoga, the practice of various modified forms of Hatha Yoga. And from that time onward, most people have associated yoga with the numerous Indian and Western schools of modern posture yoga. But, as explained above, the historical roots of yoga run much deeper and longer than that.

Tantra and Vedanta

The yoga tradition is a confluence of many metamorphosed paths, and it is often difficult to know where one path of yoga started and where it merged with another. There is also much debate about which practices are Tantric or Vedantic, or if a certain philosophical idea is from Samkhya, from the Yoga Sutras, Tantra, or Vedanta, or even whether it is a Hindu or Buddhist practice or idea. I think of it this way: the practical path of Tantra are the many expressions of yoga we find throughout history, and the various philosophies of yoga—Vedanta, Samkhya, the Yoga Sutras, Kashmir Tantra, and Bengal Tantra—are philosophical, cultural and psychological expressions created by various Tantric yogis. Some of these philosophies are nondual and others are dualistic.

I therefore like to think of yoga, Veda, Tantra, even Ayurveda, as simultaneous and interlacing paths—a religious, cultural, scientific, medical, and philosophical tapestry woven together over time. Broadly speaking, the main practical and yogic colors of this tapestry are woven from the threads of Tantra while the more religious strands stem from the four Vedas and the more subtle philosophical ones from Vedanta and Classical Yoga. But there is also a sublimely rich philosophical tradition in Tantra, especially in Kashmir Tantra, as well as in contemporary time through the composition of new Tantric sutras by teachers such as Anandamurtii.

The majority of the posture and meditation practices we essentially think of as yoga have their direct or indirect roots in Tantra—the asana practice, the mantra meditations, the yantra and chakra systems, and the basic philosophical idea of Indian philosophy, that the world is a composite of two forces—energy and consciousness, Purusha and Prakrti, or Shiva and Shakti. The latter idea is a fundamental ontological vision in most all of Indian yoga philosophy, from Samkhya to the Yoga Sutras to the various schools in the renaissance period of Tantra in the Middle Ages.

In nondual Tantra, such as in the Tantra philosophy of Abhinava Gupta and the contemporary Anandamurtii, we see the blossoming of an ecological philosophy that appeals to us modern seekers in its simple and deep brilliance: the idea that Spirit, the Divine Brahma, has two expressions, namely Shiva (Purusha) and Shakti (Prakriti), or consciousness and energy. This nondual embrace is an exquisite and unique gift of Tantric spirituality.

Tantra's Life-affirming Essence

We cannot separate Tantra from the heart of the various, ancient yogic paths and their particular history. The practice of Tantra, then, can loosely be characterized as the universal human quest for union with the Divine Source, a quest which is also found in all the other world's wisdom traditions.

Personally, I was drawn to Tantra, because of its wholesome practices and philosophy. Vedanta, on the other hand, with its more abstract philosophy, seemed too detached, ascetic and otherworldly to me. I was attracted to the Tantric embrace of both unity and duality, both wholeness and opposites.

While classical Vedanta sees the world as an illusion, in Tantra this world of opposites is real but dissolves in Brahma, in Spirit, the underlying being of all reality. And while Vedanta desires a world of detachment from the world, Tantra sees the inner essence of all life and all things as bliss and love, and that the way out of the world's entanglements is not to retreat from it but to engage with it as an expression of Brahma. To love the world. And, if necessary, to change the world. That is why Tantra is often called *the path of ecstasy*, or *the path of love*. That is why Tantra is so appealing to the environmentalist and spiritual activist in me.

Tantra's Contemporary Appeal

I think Tantra appeals to many modern yogis because of its notion that everything is Divine. This essential realization—that every form, particle, or atom of this universe has an inherent capacity to reveal the sacred; that everything is, at its core, God; that is the essence of Tantra.

Tantra appeals to us because of its alchemical use of energy, its promise to transform desire into bliss, and violence into peace. For the Tantric, all dualities, all conflicts and opposites, all forms and energies are different expressions of Brahma, and the goal of life is to ultimately dissolve in a state of nondual unity and peace. Tantra attracts the mystic in us for its adherence to nondualism; its ability to see the oneness of everything. It is perhaps this holistic and practical attitude—that Divinity is everywhere and that sacredness can be realized anywhere—that makes Tantra so appealing to us yogis in the contemporary world.

The Next Wave:
Tantric Meditation in the Yoga Studios?

There were hardly any yoga studios in Europe and the US in the early 1980s when I went to India to study Tantra. Today, yoga studios are more common than bakeries in many cities around the world. In these studios, various styles of posture yoga is performed, from Vinyasa to Yin, from Power to Ashtanga, from Iyengar to Jivamukti. There are also studios offering Chocolate Yoga, Wine Yoga, even Beer Yoga. But there are very few studios offering courses on meditation, especially yogic or Tantric meditation. But I believe this is soon about to change.

Gaia, a popular online yoga education forum, is currently offering a series of Tantric videos with Christopher Wallis featuring "micro meditations" from the Vijnana Bhairava Tantra, the text Lorin Roche made popular in the book *The Radiance Sutras*. In many yoga studios all over the world, classes end with not just chanting Om and saying Namaste with folded hands, but also with yogic and Tantric meditation.

These are all signs of a holistic tapestry being woven together from all the integrated strands of wisdom that Tantric yoga has to offer. In other words, we are presently witnessing a second reemergence of Tantra. And this time, not only in India, it is truly a global reemergence. As Westerners develop a thirst for what Tantric yoga has to offer, they will discover the vast richness of meditation practices the tradition contains. They will discover that there is more to meditation than mindfulness practices.

As yoga teacher Miles Neale says, «the health and relaxation that folks are experiencing is just the beginning.... a prelude for a much greater learning process. Yoga and meditation are capable of taking us to the moon. But if we stay at the level of Frozen Yoga and McMindfulness, it is like we are using a rocket launcher to light a candle.» (Neale, 2010)

Meditation teacher Dennis Hunter echo Neale's point by stating that "mindfulness meditation is trending these days, and is practiced everywhere from the yoga studio to the board room. But the great meditative traditions tell us that mindfulness is only a starting point. Once the mind has been tamed and trained through mindfulness, then true meditation and self-inquiry can actually begin."(Hunter, 2017)

The human thirst for a deeper and fuller yoga experience has begun, but our longing for more self-realization and transcendence will not end with Beer Yoga, nor with Chocolate Yoga. The human thirst for inner balance, for deeper soul and ecstatic spirituality is what authentic yoga has always been about, and that thirst is reflected in the next wave in yoga, and it will lead many modern yogis toward the Tantric practices of meditation and chanting that underlie all of yoga philosophy like a cool, subterranean flow of water.

Tantric Meditation Practices

In the Yoga Sutras, Patanjali explains that the last of the ten tenets of yama and niyama, the ethics of yoga, is *Ishvarapranidhana*, the practice of meditating on the Divine with love and devotion. This devotional concentration is very much at the heart of Tantric meditation, as the embrace of longing, of love as a spiritual practice. Patanjali furthermore says in the Yoga Sutras that Samadhi (the highest state of meditation) is attained by love for God or the Divine (Ishavarapranidhanadva).

In simple terms, Tantric meditation, as partly outlined in the Yoga Sutras, consists of the following practices: Pranayama, or breathing exercises, sometimes with the use of a mantra; pratyahara, or sense withdrawal, which usually consists of various visualization practices to withdraw the mind form the outside world, from the body, and then finally from feelings and thoughts; dharana, or concentration, is a practice which consists of intense focus on a chakra, sometimes combined with pranayama, silent mantra recitation and often a visualization; dhyana, or flow meditation, consists of a visualization practice without mantra that results in a real or envisioned merger in higher consciousness, in the experience of samadhi, the goal of yoga.

Proficiency in all of these meditation practices are gained through systematic, daily practice over a long period of time, and during the individual sessions when a deep, synchronized and spontaneous flow arises, when breath, mantra, meaning of the mantra, and visualizations are united in an experience of inner yoga, of union with inner consciousness.

Many scholars point out that the Yoga Sutras cannot be a Tantric text because Patanjali does not mention kundalini, the "serpent power" said to reside at the bottom of the spine, and a central aspect of Tantra. But, as we have seen above, Patanjali does include many other Tantric aspects in his famous text. Kundalini is, however, mentioned in many of the Upanishads, as amply illustrated in the comprehensive book on Laya Yoga by Shyam Sundar Goswami, thus again illustrating how Tantric teachings are scattered all throughout the yogic and Vedic texts.

In addition to the practices briefly described above, there are in Tantric yoga various chakra meditations which aims at harmonizing and strengthening the body's energy centers, and thereby also the glandular endocrine system, through the recitation of root sounds and various visualizations of geometric forms and colors.

What is the main difference between secular mindfulness meditation and yogic or Tantric meditation? The objective of mindfulness practices are to become more relaxed, peaceful, happy, and centererd. Spiritual meditation, especially yogic and Tantric meditation are often more complex to practice, and also add the infusion of spiritual vizualizations or ideations during practice, to enable an experience of oneness, of union with the goal, which, according to Patanjali and all the Tantric texts, is to experience Samadhi, spiritual union with the Divine, with Ishvara. Thus

Patanjali calls this Tantric practice «to have devotion for Ishvara.» We can thus say that there are generally two types of meditation parctices, mindfulness and concentration practice, which, when practiced together, leads to a deep sense of flow and bliss, or dhyana in Patanjali's and the Tantric systems of meditation. The state of flow resulting from concentration meditation can «bring powerful feelings of bliss and ecstasy,» writes bestselling science writer Robert Wright in his book *Why Buddhism is True*. (Wright, 2017)

Spiritual meditation is about cultivating a mindset that is absorbed in consciousness rather than in the fleeting emotions and wantings of the ego-mind. It is about seeing and feeling the divine in everything, in our body, our breath, our mantra, our chakra. As the Indian poet and sage Kabir said, "The divine is the breath inside your breath." Or, as the Sufi poet Hafiz writes in this poetic image: while meditating "become the hole in the flute that Christ's breath flows through." In this line, Hafiz exemplify the universality of all yogic, Tantric and spiritual practice—that meditation is the union between mindfulness, visualization, sound, concentration, and breath.

During the practice of pranayama, pratyahara, dharana and dhyana in Raja Yoga, Rajadhiraja Yoga, or Tantra Yoga, these spiritual metaphors inspire the yogi practitioner to go deeper in sadhana. Such lessons, however, are not an integral part of "secular" mindfulness practice.

Tantra and Yoga are One Path

There are obviously many paths of yoga. Contemporary Vinyasa is not exactly the same practice as the yoga outlined in the Hatha Yoga Pradipika of the Middle Ages. As thoroughly documented in the book *Roots of Yoga* by James Mallinson and Mark Singleton, there have been many expressions of yoga throughout the ages, many paths, many teachers.

With that I agree, but I do not agree with the many eminent

scholars who insist on separating yoga and Tantra as if they are two distinct paths, originating at different times. Broadly speaking, yoga and Tantra are, in their varied forms of practice and philosophy, expressions of a singular path for the cultivation and advancement of the body, mind, and spirit.

As I have shown above, academia, mainly due to lack of engagement as practitioners within the traditions they study, is often drawing an artificial boundary between yoga and Tantra. Yogic and Tantric culture have existed throughout the ages, and academic studies are often not reflecting the cultural and practical context in which these traditions flourished, a culture in which most teachings were oral and transmitted by teacher to student, most often without textual references at all.

To date everything in yogic and Tantric history according to texts is much like trying to date the origin of shamanism according to the time when the first Western book on the subject was written, or to date the Cherokee language according to the time when Sequoyah wrote the Cherokee alphabet in 1810. Obviously both shamanism and the Cherokee language are thousands of years older. Similarly, yoga and Tantra existed in oral form, carefully preserved in the form of sutras—short couplets containing practical, ritualistic, and philosophical knowledge—for thousands of years before they were written down as texts. Indeed, one of the main purposes of the sutra tradition was to create a system that was easy to submit to memory and pass down through time from teacher to student, from community to community.

The teachings in the Yoga Sutras are thus much older than the text itself. Moreover, they represent the author's own philosophical point of view, and often do not express or explain the yogic or Tantric practices underlying the ideas. Similarly, the various teachings in the Tantric texts from the Middle Ages are also much older and represent individual paths or gurus' idiosyncratic values and specific points of view, some of these texts, according to Anandamurtii, as old as Shiva himself. More importantly, since the yogic or Tantric techniques were held in secret and often not taught directly in the texts, it is best, if possible, to obtain knowledge from within the tradition itself, from a guru, or a teacher to learn how to practice the teachings the texts refer to.

Yoga and Tantra are like the two wings of the same bird. Broadly speaking, they have the same function and the same goal—to harmonize body, mind and spirit and through meditation to transcend the body and mind and enjoy union with the Divine within. I would not be surprised if tomorrow, as part of the evolution of everything yoga, that what we now practice as yogis and yoginis, will also be referred to as Tantra.

Chapter Three
A Brief Tantric History of Yoga

IT IS BECOMING INCREASINGLY evident that India, in so many ways, is the cradle of human civilization, not just geographically and culturally, but also spiritually. India's great civilization was born about 11,000 years ago, during or shortly after Neolithic farming settlements were established in the Fertile Crescent in the Middle East. For South Asia, including India, Pakistan and Afghanistan, was one of the first areas on the planet where people settled to farm and create urbanized city complexes on a considerable scale. In Mehrgarh, an area in today's Pakistan, wheat, barley and eggplant were cultivated, sheep and cattle were domesticated, and people lived in cities as early as nine thousand years ago. India is also the birthplace of the world's first great religions, Buddhism and Jainism. Most importantly, long before the birth of Buddha (500 BCE), India had already developed the sophisticated sciences of yoga, meditation, Ayurvedic medicine, and the world's most advanced and sacred language, Sanskrit.

While there is general agreement among scholars regarding the antiquity of India's civilization, there is less agreement about how and when it developed its sophisticated culture and sacred traditions. There are currently three main theories on ancient Indian history:

1. Many Western and Indian academics still subscribe to the view that India was invaded by Vedic Aryan settlers around 1900 BCE. These Aryans worshiped the sun god Suria and brought with them their Rigvedic religion based on sacrifices and rituals offered to "placate and please the Gods, [and] to force them to fulfill wishes

and demands." (Dieter-Stuhl, 2000) These patriarchal and martial Aryans soon conquered northern India and destroyed the great Indus Valley civilization, where yoga was already practiced by Tantric ascetics. They massacred populations and reduced the surviving Dravidian *shudras* to slavery (dasyu) without regard for rank or learning. This conflict has been described in the famous epics Mahabharata and the Ramayana. Over time, India became a blended civilization—part Aryan Vedic, part Dravidian Shaiva, with a liberal admixture of Jain and Buddhist traditions—and this blended culture is what we today know as Hindu civilization.

2. Western yoga scholars, including Georg Feuerstein and David Frawley, as well as some Indian writers, especially within the Hindutva movement, subscribe to the theory that there was never an Aryan invasion around 1900 BCE and that yoga comes solely from the Vedic tradition. I call this the One River Theory. Rather than being destroyed by nomadic warriors, the Indus Valley civilization, they claim, was destroyed and abandoned due to climatic changes. According to these writers, the Aryans are indigenous to India and represent everything that is noble about Indian culture. In the book *In Search of the Cradle of Civilization*, Feuerstein and Frawley outline 17 points for why the invasion never took place. In one of these points, however, they reflect on the possibility that the Aryan settlers arrived in India at a much earlier date. This alternative idea is, of course, exactly what I am proposing in this book.

3. The real history of yoga, therefore, represents a blend of the Tantric and Vedic traditions of India. Since both Puranic history as well as genetic science suggest that the Vedic Aryans arrived in India at an early age, most likely as early as 5000 BCE, the blending of the Vedic and Tantric cultures of India had already matured by the time the Indus Valley civilization was destroyed and depopulated around 2000 BCE. Not long after, around 1500

BCE, India produced the world's first coherent philosophy and cosmology, namely sage Kapila's Tantric-inspired Samkhya philosophy, which today is popularly known as the philosophy of Ayurveda, India's ancient medical science. About 700 years after Kapila, some of the greatest spiritual literature the world has ever witnessed, namely the oral teachings in the epic Mahabharata, the Vedantic Upanishads, the spiritual teachings of the Gita, and the historical mythology of the Ramayana were written down for the first time. And around 200 BCE, sage Patanjali wrote his Yoga Sutras and codified the oral teachings of the Tantric yogis for the first time in the form of Asthanga, or Raja Yoga.

While these three broad versions of Indian history may seem entirely at odds, there are important overlapping agreements, and the theories do in many ways compliment each other. The first theory has dated the Aryan invasion rather late (1900 BCE) and does not reflect the genetic research of Dr. Spencer Wells, who, as mentioned in the introduction, claims the migration may have started before 5000 BCE. As suggested as a possibility by Feuerstein and Frawley—proponents of theory number two—this invasion thus took place when the Rigvedic Aryans arrived via the Russian steppes and the deserts of Iran about 3000 years before the Indus Valley eventually was abandoned. Looking for better pastures for their cattle, and for other riches, these skilled warrior nomads arrived in successive raids and migrations over a period of several millennia. They arrived in an already inhabited land, and its peoples—the Dravidians, Mongolians and Austrics—had already developed a sophisticated, urban culture, and the art and science of Tantric Yoga was already in practice among them. In other words, by the time the Indus Valley was finally abandoned, the indigenous Indians and the invading Aryans had already experienced 3000 years of conflict and gradual integration. Hence these two peoples, representing two different civilizations, cultures and outlooks—one priestly and one yogic—gradually formed what we know today as the Indian, or Hindu Civilization.

A Very Brief History of Tantra: The Two River Theory

In his award-winning book, *A Brief History of India*, Alain Danielou outlines in broad, colorful strokes an ancient history of India that contrasts with the one presented to most Western yoga students, who are often told Tantra and yoga originated in the Vedas. Danielou reminds us, however, that yoga originated with the ancient sage Shiva and that these practices were "wholly unknown" to the early Vedas and their authors, the invading Aryans. (Danielou, 2003)

Danielou is not alone in this assertion. According to multiple sources, it was the Shiva Tantrics who taught the early Indians yogic spirituality, the arts and sciences. Moreover, these Shiva teachings, remained the dominant culture and spiritual teachings in India, even though its adherents were often violently attacked by the early Vedic Aryans. The Tantric teachings of Shiva continued to be the religion of the people, Danielou asserts, and what we today have come to appreciate as Indian spiritual culture and religion was more influenced by Tantra than the Vedas. This assertion, which will be emphasized in this book, is contrary to what most modern yogis are taught about the history of their practice.

Danielou also emphasizes the importance of Shiva Tantra in shaping yoga philosophy, culture and practice. "It should be remembered," he writes, "that in Hinduism, Yoga is a discipline created by Shiva..." (Danielou, 2003) From early on, the culture and spiritual practices that originated with Shiva's Tantra also spread outside India, even as far as Europe. Writes Danielou: "Although—due to scarcity of documentation—the importance of this great fundamental religion in the formation of later religions has been largely under-estimated, it was almost universal."(Danielou, 2003)

Vikings and Tantrics

Long before I knew anything about Tantra and ancient Indian history, I met a traveler and writer from Norway, my native country. He had just returned from an adventurous trip to Afghanistan, Nepal and India. Inspired by American spiritual seekers, most notably well-known psychologist and author Ram Dass and popular beat poet Allen Ginsberg, he was one of the first Europeans to visit these countries by traveling over land through Turkey, Iran and Iraq. His name was Eivind Reinertsen, and he told remarkable tales from his many trips to the East. He published a landmark book called *Journey Without Arrival (Reise Uten Ankomst*, Aschehoug Forlag) about these travels, and a few years later, he became an award-winning poet.

I met Reinertsen during a visit to some student friends living in an alternative community in Oslo. My friends had recently learned transcendental meditation (TM), so our conversation that night focused mainly on their newfound practice. Our topic quickly changed, however, when Reinertsen suddenly made a startling claim. He said there had been a secret society of Tantric yogis on the west coast of Norway during the Viking era (ca. 800-1200 CE). Although I have never been able to verify this rather fantastic historical possibility, there are interesting clues scattered about in Viking history that makes Reinertsen's claim seem at least remotely probable.

The Vikings were not exactly renowned for their peaceful and introspective ways, so the story seemed a bit far-fetched, and I was reluctant to believe him. But his story did pique my interest in yoga. Shortly thereafter, I began reading about the mysterious world of Tantra—its philosophy, history, and especially its yogic practices. A few years later, after having lived in a yoga ashram in Copenhagen, Denmark, for a couple of years, I decided to go to India in order to immerse myself fully in the study and lifestyle of Tantra Yoga.

Pashupati:
The Tantric God Who Traveled the World

Some time after I met Reinertsen, I was reminded of his fantastic stories by a photo I discovered of a bronze sculptured yogi sitting in lotus pose on a "bucket" found on the *Oseberg*, Norway's most famous and best preserved ship from the Viking era. In the summer of 2005, I visited the Viking museum in Oslo to see this remarkable bucket with my own eyes. This so-called "Buddha bucket" is a wooden pail made of strips of yew held together with brass bands. The "ears" to which the handle is attached depicts two yogic brass figures sitting in lotus position with closed eyes. Prominently displayed on the chests of these two meditating yogis are four swastikas or "hakekors," as the Vikings called these sacred symbols. The swastika, a symbol of spiritual victory in Tantra, has been in existence in India since the time of Shiva, but is also known as a scared symbol among the Vikings, the Greeks as well as the Egyptians. In fact, the swastika is a symbol of Shiva and Shakti and is often prominently displayed on houses and temples all over Asia. Unfortunately, the Nazis misused this deeply spiritual symbol for their evil purposes.

What could be the origin of this "meditating Viking"? Such practices could have originated from the contact Europeans had with Asian people during the migration times. On the other hand, the technique could have been known among Celtic and Germanic people, passed down since the time of Shiva. It is also possible, but less likely, thesemeditation practices developed independently by Nordic shamans. Shamanic elements are well known in the North Germanic religionsas well as inmost native cultures all over the world. We also know that the term "útisetia" (literally "sitting outside"), from ancient Norse literature, indicates a "trance technique" that could indeed refer to yogic meditation. We know for certain that the practice of sitting in the lotus position is not common among shamanic cultures. Hence, it is very likely the Buddha Bucket illustrates a Viking practicing yogic meditation. Metallurgic experts believe the figure has been made locally, since a similarly made standing figure has been found at Myklebostad in Norway.

Not long after I encountered the Buddha Bucket figure, I learned about the Gundesrup Cauldron (400-100 BCE), a silver bowl found in a peat bog in Denmark. This famous artifact appears to depict the image of Pashupati, or Shiva. The image of the alleged Shiva on the Gundesrup Cauldron is strikingly similar to the many seals attributed to Shiva found in the Indus Valley during the archaeological digs by Sir John Marshall between 1922 and 1931. Commonly known as a place were Tantra was widely practiced, this great culture, located at the archaeological site of Harappa and Mohenjo-Daro (4000-2000 BCE), is as old and as sophisticated as the ancient civilization of Mesopotamia. At the time, these and the other rice-growing areas of Asia boasted a concentration of approximately one-quarter of the world's population.

In the famous seals found at Harappa and Mohenjo-Daro, Shiva sits in a yogic posture allowing the back to remain comfortably erect and thus to make it easier to concentrate during meditation. His feet are formed into an advanced Tantric practice that forms a lock under the genital area and thus helps direct psychic energy up through the spine. On the Gundestrup Cauldron, however, the Shiva figure sits in a different posture, in the "easy pose," also commonly used for meditation practice.

During my monastic training in India the 1980s, I became intimately familiar with Pashupati—the Lord of the Beasts. It happened while I spent time alone as a *sadhu*, meditating and begging for my food near Pashupatinat, a Shiva temple located in the small town of Deopatan, to the east of Kathmandu. This ancient temple is a major destination for Hindu pilgrims from all over India and Nepal. It is situated to the south of a gorge carved out by the Bagmati River. Pashupatinat, often crowded by both pious pilgrims and wild monkeys, resides by the river, above the sacred funeral *ghats* where the dead are cremated daily on top of large piles of burning wood.

Snaking along the Pashupatinat temple walls, the Bagmati is considered as sacred as the Ganges itself. For Hindus, to bathe at Pashupatinat on particular phases of the moon is to ensure a place in Shiva's Paradise, Kailash. For Tantric yogis, however, all rivers and places are sacred, and Shiva's Paradise is to be realized within each yogi's own heart, not in some distant place in the afterlife or at a sacred site.

Like the Indus Valley seal, the Nepali temple is dedicated to Pashupati. Pashu means "beast," or "animal," so the esoteric meaning of Pashupati in Tantra is "the controller of animal instincts." In other words, in order to become free, we must redirect and become free from our instinctual tendencies, our psychological bondages. According to yoga, there are eight bondages, or *asthapashas*, which includes fear, shyness, doubt, pride of heritage, pride of culture, vanity, and backbiting, as well as the six enemies or *sadripus*, which includes lust, rage, greed, attachment to objects, pride, and envy. Lord Pashupati is thus a symbol of someone who has overcome these inner beasts, and Tantric yoga is a spiritual path whose ultimate goal is to overcome, or not be controlled by, these "wild beasts" of the mind.

Embracing the Wild Beasts of the Mind

In the evening, that first day at Pashupatinat, I was walking by the river, careful not to step on meditating or sleeping yogis. I noticed a group of half-naked bodies sitting in a circle around a towering figure with long, matted hair and beard. He was seated, like Shiva himself, in lotus pose. A few of his words, drifting in the smoke-filled breeze, caught my attention. "Astapasha and sadripu…" Then he recited them, first the eight bondages— *bhaya, ghr'na, lajja, shamka, kula, shiila, mana, yugupsa.* Then the six enemies, *kama, krodha, lobha, moha, mada, matsarya.* The ancient Sanskrit flowed out of him like poetry. And even though I did not understand the Hindi commentary that followed, I sat down to join the small circle of yogis around the glowing embers from the dying fire. After some time, the yogi on the tiger skin became silent. His eyes of piercing kindness looked into mine for a moment. Then, oblivious to the chatter and commotion among the pilgrims along the river, he closed his eyes and began to meditate.

A few days later, I walked down a street near the temple toward the fireplace where I prepared my one meal for the day. My cotton shoulder bag contained two potatoes, a handful of rice, a few coins, some matches and one red chili. The meager collection from my begging round that morning was not unusual. Most shopkeepers thought it rather unlikely that I, Westerner, could be a wandering *sadhu*, a true holy man. Thinking I was a fraud, they often refused to give me anything. They were partly right, of course. As part of my monastic training, I was a wandering beggar, but only for a while, not for life.

An old woman, a real beggar, suddenly stopped me on the street and held out her hand. I was not allowed to speak during my begging period, so I gestured with my hands that I did not have anything to give her. My answer did not satisfy her. She became very angry, waved with her hands and pointed at my tan yet unmistakably white skin. Obviously, she was unable to tell that I also was a beggar, even if only temporarily. To her, I was simply a "rich Westerner." So, I gave her my last few coins, which I usually used to buy matches and cooking oil with. Not satisfied, she threw them on the ground and spat on them. Disappointed, I asked her to open her own bag, and I emptied my own bag of goods into hers. Potatoes, rice, chili, matches, coins—all my money and my one and only meal for the day—it all disappeared into the old beggar's dilapidated bag. That, I thought, was a truly benevolent act. I had given up all my food for that day to an old woman, a beggar for life. I was proud of myself for accomplishing such a great act of unselfish service, despite my rather meager condition.

After the old woman looked into her bag, she became more furious. She was truly insulted. How could I, a rich Westerner, give her so little? She stomped her bare feet; she spat; she held up the two potatoes. Then she threw both of them on the ground and walked away.

My inner beasts, especially the fetters of pride and rage, were cruelly awakened that day. When I finally succumbed to my day of hunger and meditation, and my anger subsided, I was humbled, truly humbled. I had yet to learn the art of true selflessness, to give the gift of love and compassion without expecting anything in return. But since Tantra teaches us that our problems are our best friends, I eventually learned to look at that old, angry beggar as a great friend and teacher.

Tantra and Ayurveda

A few years before my journey to India and Nepal, I received my initiation in Tantra meditation at a retreat in a pine forest in Sweden by a Tantric monk in saffron robes who had recently arrived from India. In accordance with ancient tradition, the charismatic monk whispered a mantra into my right ear and told me it was never to be uttered aloud, except back to him. He prescribed a specific technique for withdrawing my mind from its external preoccupations, guiding it away from attachment to the body, and meditating on and become one with the mantra's deep meaning. I was to recite the mantra silently, in harmony with my breath, while concentrating on a particular *chakra*. This first of the six lessons I was to learn in Tantric meditation seemed a bit complicated at first, but I soon got the hang of it. Indeed, I experienced some very powerful visions and spiritual insights at that very first retreat. I had found my spiritual home, and ever since that gathering, I have practiced Tantric meditation daily.

Later on that auspicious day, I heard several stories about Shiva, not the well known Hindu deity, but the historical Shiva, a living person who, like the Buddha, was an enlightened yogi. According to the oral history of the Tantric tradition, it was he who systematized Tantra Yoga and who also enhanced Vaedyak Shastra, the ancient system of yogic or Tantric medicine, which is basically the same as what we today know as Ayurveda. It is common knowledge among Ayurvedic doctors in Nepal and India that there is a historical and spiritual interrelationship between Tantra and Ayurveda. Furthermore, when I was in India, I was taught that Shiva was the preceptor of the first group of Ayurvedacharyas, or the teachers of Ayurveda.

When I studied Ayurveda at the California College of Ayurveda, a school that maintains that Ayurveda is a Vedic science only, I learned that Lord Dhanvantari was "the God of Ayurveda and of healing." Lord Dhanvantari is said to have been a high- caste king of Benares, which during Shiva's time was called Kashi, and who taught an Ayurvedic form of surgery. From a Tantric perspective, it makes sense that Dhanvantari taught surgery because that was part of the science of Tantric Ayurveda. Dhanvantari could not have been a follower of the Vedas, however, since Vedic dogmas prohibited high-caste Brahmins to touch people of a lower caste, and thus prohibited them from performing surgery. As it is said in the oral tradition of Tantra, it is more likely to conclude that Dhanvantari was a Tantric and also Shiva's first and main apprentice in Ayurveda. In other words, as Anandamurti claims, Dhanvantari was most likely the world's first Ayurvedic teacher.

Contemporary Ayurvedic writers, including Deepak Chopra, David Frawley and Vasant Lad, have, in their books, revealed some of the sublime wisdom found in Ayurvedic medical texts, including the famed *Carakasamhita*. Yet these popular writers have overlooked the fact that Ayurveda's ancient roots also trail back to Tantric teachings passed down through the ages since Shiva's time.

Tantric and Ayurvedic Medical Science in Ancient India

According to Ayurveda, disease occurs when the balance of the body is lost due to an increase or decrease of the body's three humors—*vata, pitta or kapha*. Medicine is applied to restore balance. If the amount of vata or pitta decreases, medicine is applied to increase it; if the amount of vata or pitta increases, medicine is applied to decrease it. This, in simple terms, is the Ayurvedic system of medicine.

Rudimentary forms of Ayurveda were, according to Anandamurtii, brought to India by the Aryan people as early as 8-7,000 years ago. About 7,000 years ago, Shiva further developed the Tantric system of medicine that incorporated and refined Ayurveda. This new, advanced system of medicine also included surgery. For thousands of years, the Indian medical system was a mixture of these two schools of medicine—Tantric and Vedic. Thus, in the Ayurvedic teachings popularized today, it is difficult to distinguish which feature is Tantric and which is Vedic. (Anandamurtii, 1994)

During the age of the Mahabharata, about 1500 BCE, surgery, Ayurveda, Vaedyak Shastra, and even a rudimentary form of homeopathy existed in India. During that time, Lord Krishna developed another branch of medicine called Visa Cikitsa. Due to certain Vedic religious dogmas, however, the Tantric science of surgery was largely discontinued because it was forbidden to touch dead bodies.

From the ancient Tantric seers, we have learned there were eight main branches of medicine, which form the basis of the eight main divisions of Ayurveda:

1. Salya Tantra: Healing of wounds in the lower limbs through surgery.
2. Salakya Tantra: Healing of wounds in the upper limbs through surgery.

3. Kayacikitsa Tantra: Healing of internal and external diseases.
4. Bhutavidya Tantra: Healing of mental diseases.
5. Kaumarabhritia Tantra: Healing of children's diseases.
6. Agada Tantra: The science of toxicology.
7. Vajikarana Tantra: The science of sexual balance and vigor.
8. Rasayana Tantra: The science of rejuvenation.

In Ayurvedic books today, we learn that the medical source for this ancient science is a book called the *Carakasamhita*. This book, however, is actually a revised version of an earlier work called *Agnivesa Tantra*, written by the Tantric sage AgZnivesa. These ancient Tantric yogis were also skilled in the art of alchemy and, much like today's homeopaths, used many altered toxic substances, including mercury, for healing and transformation. In Tantra, the body is seen as the microcosm of the universe. Longevity and health are thus achieved through spiritual union with Cosmic Consciousness and in living in harmony with the complex, yet orderly, natural forcesin the cosmos within and beyond us.

Did Shiva Travel to Europe?

In 1979, I had another pivotal experience in my understanding of Tantric history. It occurred during my meeting with the guru, Shrii Shrii Anandamurtii. An enigmatic person who allegedly could read people's present and past lives as if they were books. Anandamurtii was also hailed as "one of the greatest philosophers of modern India" by former Indian President Giani Zail Singh. Already well known in India with a fast-growing group of devoted followers, he had embarked upon a whirlwind tour to nine countries on four continents.

After a few days of listening to this electrifying and mysterious man's lectures and watching people fall in yogic trance, or *samadhi*, around him, I found myself walking beside him with a group of people along a mountain road in the beautiful Fiesch valley in

Switzerland. Once in a while, the guru would stop, point toward
a flower I had never seen or toward an unusual shrub and explain
in detail these plants' local and Latin names, their medicinal properties and the kind of soil they best thrived in. At other times, he
would pick up a rock and give a lengthy description of its various
mineral properties, or he would point toward a picturesque farm
far away and explain in great detail what kind of fruit crops the
farmer cultivated and what other types of crops would be good
to grow in that area. His encyclopedic knowledge of everything
around us was simply breathtaking, especially since he had never
before been to that part of the world.

On one of these walks, with another group of people, Anandamurtii suddenly stopped and looked out across the snow-covered
Swiss Alps and exclaimed that Shiva traveled from India to this
valley about 7,000 years ago on a yak.

During his European trip in 1979, Anandamurti also made some
predictions about the future. While standing besides the infamous
Berlin Wall, which at that time still divided West Germany from
East Germany, Western democracy from Eastern Communism, he
said, "This wall symbolizes the brutal suppression by Communism
against human liberties. It is a kind of artificial madness. In the
near future, you will see this wall crumble piece by piece, stone by
stone. East and West Germany will be united as one."

As predicted, this historical unification occurred 10 years later,
in 1989. Two years earlier, in 1987, Anandamurtii made another
prediction about the future by saying that Communism would
soon "fall like a house of cards." Indeed, it did—in 1989, in country after country, Communism disappeared in Eastern Europe.

I have often wondered, is it not conceivable--that this mystic seer
and sage, who could read people, rocks and plants as if they were
books, who could see into the future as if it happened before him-
-that he could also, with equal accuracy, see into and explain the
past? As we have already learned, genetic science has now proved
he was right in his prediction about the Aryan migration into India.

When a Tantric yogi, through psycho-spiritual practice, makes his mind as expansive as the Comic Mind, he can receive information directly from that Source. This is sometimes referred to as the *akashic records,* a cosmic storehouse of information and knowledge, easily accessible to psychics and clairvoyant yogis. In other words, by mentally accessing this subtle field of consciousness. According to yogic epistemology, it is thus possible for a great yogic master to reveal the secrets of both the past and the future.

So, if Shiva, the father of Tantra indeed left his Himalayan abode to travel all the way to Europe, one might assume that some of the Tantric teachings also took root in the rocky soil of the Swiss Alps and from there ventured beyond. In accordance with my Norwegian author friend, as well as Dr. John Mumford and Alain Danielou, both scholars and yogic adepts who have written about the ancient interconnection between pagan and yogic history, Tantra, at least in mythological form, could thus have spread toward the Celts in Germany, France and the British Isles and even farther north toward the Bronze Age farmers and Vikings of Scandinavia.

Tracing Tantra from the Roots

India is an enormous country with a long and culturally rich history. In the past, it has included Pakistan, Bangladesh, Afghanistan, Burma, and Sri Lanka. Perhaps the most ancient civilization on the planet, India has an uncanny ability both to move beyond and embrace its past. And, more often than not, this multifaceted country mirrors the vastness, depth and history of humanity itself.

Indian civilization may not only be the planet's oldest continuous civilization, but also the one with the richest and most enduring spiritual legacy. According to Anandamurtii, basic forms of Tantra existed even prior to Shiva's time, leaving a trail back to early shamanic cultures. In fact, he once directed some of my yogi friends to a cave in Northeastern India where they discovered depictions of the esoteric yogic chakra system painted, in graphic detail, on the cave walls. These cave paintings, he claims, are nearly 9,000 years old.

In India, I was taught that the earliest systematic Tantric teachings are formulated in the Agama and Nigama Tantras. These esoteric teachings are allegedly based on conversations between Shiva and his wife Parvati. The Nigama teachings constitute the philosophical teachings of Tantra, or the deeply inquisitive questions that Parvati posed to Shiva. The Agama teachings make up the practical aspects, or the answers that Shiva gave.

The more I delved into Anandamurti's teachings, I realized how Tantra had influenced the Vedas, including the Upanishads, which were written after the four Vedas. This iso-called Fifth Veda includes many references to Tantric concepts, such as the subtle life-force energies, or *vayus,* and the psychic energy vortexes today commonly known as *chakras.* Most importantly, the deep philosophy of the Upanishads flourished in a culture steeped in Tantric practice. "The Tantric esprit," writes Feuerstein, "continues to evolve through the period of the Brahmanas and Upanishads (ca. 2000 BCE), as well as the intellectually and spiritually fertile era of the Mahabharata, until it reached its typical form in the Tantras of the early common era." (Feuerstein, 1998) In the ensuing centuries, Tantra experienced a booming renaissance, and its philosophy and practices had a remarkable influence on Tibetan Buddhism, Hinduism, as well as the lesser known Jainism.

The age-old spiritual science of Tantra is as timely as ever. Within its vast synthesis of spiritual cosmology and yogic techniques, you will find all the required knowledge to achieve physical, mental and spiritual balance. Tantra's integral approach to life—for Tantra sees our human body, mind and spirit as a microcosmic mirror of the cosmos itself—is especially relevant to all those who appreciate the value of a spiritual and sustainable lifestyle.

Dispelling Some Myths about Yoga and Tantra

Although many Vedic priests also practiced Tantra, due to their own prejudices, they attempted to demonstrate the Vedic origin of Tantra and yoga. One may find an example of such misrepresentation in the Rudrayamala Tantra, where it is said that "The science which comes from the mouth of Lord Shiva, goes to the ears of Parvati, and is approved by Lord Krishna, is called Agama." As Anandamurti has pointed out, however, it is illogical that Krishna of the Mahabharata era (1500 BCE) would approve something that Shiva said 3500 years earlier. This aphorism, Anandamurti asserts, "was cleverly included in the Rudrayamala Tantra by the protagonists of the Vedas."

Arthur Avalon (a.k.a. Sir John Woodroffe), the famous British writer on Tantra, spent half his life searching for secretly guarded Tantric texts in India. In his path-breaking book on the chakras and the kundalini, *The Serpent Power,* published in 1918, he also traced the origins of Tantra back to the Vedas. Avalon, as well as many other eminent Western writers on Tantra and yoga today, vehemently proclaims the Vedic origins of Tantra. They do not explain, however, why Tantric spirituality in India has long been considered *Vedabhaya*, an inferior path that belongs outside the Vedas. While we may excuse these Western writers for their ignorance, history speaks for itself: for several millennia, the followers of Tantra faced ridicule and suppression, its practices have been misunderstood, and its origin as the source of yoga either ignored or forgotten.

Despite these misgivings, Avalon is unparalleled in his comprehensive understanding of Tantra. More importantly, for those on the spiritual path, Avalon reminds us that Tantric spirituality "has the supreme merit of accomplishing within a short time what other methods can hardly accomplish within a life."

Yoga Journal, the world's most popular yoga magazine, has also perpetuated the myth that the history of yoga and Tantra started in the Vedic period. One of this magazine's regular contributors, Linda Sparrowe, writes that the history of yoga started in the Vedic Period (1500 BCE), continued to grow in the Pre-classical period (800-500 BCE), was systematized by Patanjali in the Classical Period (200 BCE), and has continued to develop into our times.

She writes that "Tantra emerged early in the post-classical period, around the fourth century C.E., but didn't reach its full flowering until 500 to 600 years later." She concludes that, for most students of yoga today, Tantra "represents a rather radical departure for yoga philosophy." In the same Magazine, Maria Carrico writes that the Vedas, India's ancient religious texts, gave birth to both the literature and the technique of yoga. These writers thus continue to perpetuate the myths about Tantra so prevalent among writers, teachers and students of yoga today.

Veda and Tantra:
The Two Spiritual Rivers of India

When studying Tantra in India, I found such bias to be quite common among Vedic scholars. Many of the Tantric teachers and scholars I met, however, explained that Tantra developed in the pre-Vedic period when it was popular among the Dravidians and the Mongolians and to a lesser extent among the Austrics. It was during this time, Shiva's authority as Tantric yogi, spiritual preceptor, medical scientist and musician emerged.

It is impossible for us to fully measure the comprehensive nature of Shiva's influence today, but it appears that Shiva was not only the "King of the Yogis" but also the leader of many tribal groups. Thus, as popularly accepted in India, none other than this Tantric yogi, deserves the term "father of yoga" as well as "father of Indian civilization."

That said, I also discovered that there are many philosophical similarities between Vedic and Tantric teachings. This similarity you will especially discover in many Sanskrit verses from the Vedas and the Tantras. In the Vedas, it is said:

Yato va ima›ni bhu›tani
Ja'yante yena ja'ta'ni jiivanti
Yatprayantyabhisam'vishanti
Tadvijijina'sasva tadbrahma.

All created beings emerge, are maintained and finally dissolve in the flow of Cosmic ideation. Make an attempt to know that Supreme Entity, the veritable Brahma.

In Tantra, a similar idea has been expressed:

Yato vishvam' samudbhu'tam' yenaja'tainca tis't'hati
Yasmin sarva'n'i liiyante jinayam' tadbrahmalaks'aen'aeh.

The entity in whom the creation, preservation and destruction of the universe takes place is Brahma.

Both the Vedic and Tantric teachings are in philosophical agreement that Brahma, the Cosmic Consciousness, is the all-pervading source of all creation. Moreover, both paths believe that the goal of life is to realize this infinite source. So, what has been the most obvious difference between Vedic and Tantric teachings? Its practices. While Tantrics meditate and practice yoga asanas, the Vedic Brahmin priests chant hymns and offer ablutions to the sacrificial fires. Since many Vedic Aryans practiced Tantra, however, over time, these two distinct streams of Indian culture have fed and nourished each other.

In one of his many discourses, Anandamurtii said that it has been Tantra, and to a lesser extent the Vedas, that has been the sacred thread holding the colorful fabric of Indian society together. Indians have always been a deeply spiritual people, and Tantra has been part and parcel of their daily life since the early dawn of civilization. While in India, I saw firsthand how Tantric culture is expressed through the devotion people have for such popular deities as Kali, Durga and Shiva. An especially popular practice is the age-old worship of the Shiva *lingam* and the *yoni,* ancient male and female fertility figures.

The lingam and yoni were originally worshiped by the early fertility cults. But over time, these sacred stones were infused with Tantric esoteric meaning. The male lingam represents Shiva, or Cosmic Consciousness, and the female yoni represents Shakti, or Cosmic Energy, of the Tantric cosmology. In other words, the lingam is the masculine Shiva, and the yoni is the feminine Shakti principles of creation. Merged together in union, they are the two faces of Brahma—the sublime fusion of duality that dissolves in Cosmic nonduality.

But what is the main reason why so many believe Tantra came from the Vedas? First, the *Tantra Shastras*—the Tantric writings of the early Common Era—were, to some extent, influenced by Vedic philosophy. Second, the Vedas were also influenced by the Tantras, because many, if not most of the Vedic sages and philosophers, including the famous Vedantic yogi and philosopher Shankara-charya (788-822 CE), were Tantric adepts. Why? Because it was Tantra, not the Vedic teachings, that contained the more practical and sophisticated wisdom and techniques needed to attain spiritual enlightenment. It is namely within the Tantric heritage that one will find the time-tested tools to become an accomplished yogi or yogini, including the esoteric sciences of *kundalini* awakening, yogic breathing, yoga exercises, and mantra meditation.

In summary, Tantra influenced the Vedas and the Vedas influenced Tantra. However, it is the Tantric path that is most responsible for the teachings we today commonly know and practice as yoga and meditation.

In the insightful book, *History of Mysticism*, S. Abhayananda reveals the story of humanity's recurrent experience of enlightenment in various cultures throughout the ages. To him, it appears that the Dravidyan civilization was based on a "full-blown Shiva-Shakti mythology" and that we therefore may trace the Tantric and Yogic tradition back to pre-Aryan India.

As Anandamurtii has repeatedly stated, all authentic yoga practice is based on Tantra. And Shiva, according to Danielou, "is the Central figure of pre-Aryan Dravidian religion in India and in all its branches in the Near East and around the Mediterranean, as far as pre-Celtic Europe." Danielou further claims that Shiva Tantra at one point was "almost universal" and has maintained its original form in India until today. The widespread veneration of Shiva in prehistoric times—from the banks of the Ganges to the shores of Europe— may explain the legends and sculptures of Viking yogis, puts in perspective Shiva's seal found in a Bronze Age peat bog in Denmark, makes it possible that Shiva traveled all the way to the Alps, and might be the source for why the Greeks speak of India as the sacred homeland of Dionysus. (Danielou, 1987)

Chapter Four
Dravidians and Aryans:
Cultural Clash and Integration

M OST CONTEMPORARY YOGA SCHOLARS maintain that Tantra as a spiritual path has virtually disappeared from India. Tantra is practiced only in Tibet in the form of Tantric Buddhism, they maintain. Moreover, many Indians think of Tantra as black magic and that it only exists on the periphery of Indian culture, among magicians and obscure sects of naked sadhus. But nothing could be farther from the truth. The teachings of Shiva flows like a subterranean river throughout most of Indian culture.

Since Shiva's time, Tantra has been widespread in India and other parts of the world in broadly two ways— as a culture and devotional practice for the common people, and as a sophisticated yogic path. Although the vast majority of Indians do not practice the more esoteric aspects of Tantra Yoga, Tantra is alive and well in India today as a way of life, as religious myth, and as a devotional source of inspiration. "The Hindu religion, as it is practiced today," writes Danielou, is tantric in character, based almost exclusively on the Agama(s)....If we wish to understand Indian thought, we must return to its sources...the Shaiva religion, the cosmological theory called Samkhya, the practices of Yoga, as well as the bases of what we consider to be Hindu philosophy, are part." (Danielou, 1987)

While only a small percentage of Indians are engaged in Tantric meditation practice, Tantric Bhakti Yoga, as spiritual practices and ways of life, is very popular and has the same ancient roots, namely the teachings of Shiva and Krishna. Krishna lived in India around 1500 BCE and advanced the idea of Bhakti Yoga, the yoga of devotion. Krishna also introduced the concepts of Karma Yoga, the yoga of action, and Jnana Yoga, the yoga of knowledge, and he emphasized, in typical Tantric style, the importance of maintaining balance between these three paths of spirituality. And from these two great personalities, Shiva and Krishna, Tantra has spread, transformed and inspired Indian society over thousands of years.

Hence, it is fair to say that Tantra is widely recognized and practiced in India today, not only in India, but throughout the world. Indeed, even in the most commercialized and body-centered yoga studios in Hollywood, various forms of Tantra Yoga are practiced, since Hatha Yoga was actually developed by Shiva Tantrics. Bhakti Yoga, the yoga of devotion—from idol worship to devotional *bhajans* and *kirtans*—is also an expression of Tantra. This form of ecstatic, trance-induced worship is widely practiced in India today. In the West, especially in the US, kirtan and bhajan concerts have also become popular among practitioners of yoga and meditation, thanks, in part, to kirtan singers like Jai Uttal and Krishna Das.

In India, many worshipers pray to the physical form of a deity rather than directly to Spirit beyond form. While this kind of idol worship is considered a style of meditation or *sadhana* in Tantra, it is acknowledged as a rudimentary style. The practical and liberal path of Tantra simply recognizes that not all people have the inclination or time to engage in sophisticated meditation techniques or practice advanced yoga postures.

One of my favorite Indian saints, Paramahansa Ramakrishna, was also one of the most prominent and beloved Tantric gurus in India in the 19th century. Famous for his worship of the image of Mother Kali, an expression of Shakti, Ramakrishna worshipped this Divine Creative Principle both day and night. His spiritual fixation or devotion to Mother Kali was so strong that he often could be seen talking to her as if she were a real person. From Ramakrishna, we thus learn one of the most important lessons of Tantra: The objective world of duality and form is, for the saints, nothing but nondual Divinity, nothing but pure Consciousness. Ramakrishna's devotion teaches us that the image of the Mother, or any image of the Beloved, is the form that can open our hearts to the formless bliss of yogic union with the Divine. For in Tantra, through the fixation of mind on a deity, a mantra, yantra, or the image of the guru, we can transcend form altogether and ecstatically reach mystical union with Spirit. We will then realize the deep, inner essence of Tantra— that all forms are a continuum of Cosmic Consciousness.

Praising the Divine through devotional songs and chants is commonly practiced by millions of people in India. This Bhakti Yoga practice is considered one of the most refined forms of Tantra. Once, I experienced this simple yoga of joyous rapture while walking down a quiet street in Kathmandu at night. After strolling down the narrow dirt road, I ended up at an open square with a small pavilion in the middle. Upon the circular platform, a group of about a dozen men sat around singing devotional bhajans to the accompaniment of a drum and a harmonium. There was no one else around. Obviously, they did not sing to entertain, earn money or seek fame. They simply sang because of their love for God. Although I did not understand much of what they sang that night, I walked away deeply touched by their effortless hymns of ecstatic devotion.

No one group of people embodies the spirit of Tantric Bhakti Yoga more than the Baul singers of Bengal. These wandering minstrels, whom I sometimes encountered on my travels in Bengal, have always lived beyond the narrow confines of religion. Their philosophy and tradition of devotional chanting grew out of the culture surrounding the Jain Tantrics of the middle ages. Their culture was also greatly influenced by the Bhakti Yoga in the Vaesnava Tantra movement of Caetanya Mahaprabhu, who lived around 1100 CE. Clad in flowing robes, strumming a one-stringed *ektar*, the Bauls have long been an integral part of Bengal's lush cultural landscape, wandering from village to village singing of a universal God. Their message of spiritual love has also crossed the borders of India since many of the songs composed by popular American kirtan performer Jai Uttal are inspired by the enchanted Baul singers. But, unfortunately, the Bauls, like many Tantrics in the past, are often perceived as heretics and still sometimes experience persecution from fundamentalist Muslims and Hindus.

Tantra—An Indian Way of Life

In India, among poor and rich, in cities and in remote villages, I often encountered a simple celebration of life. This celebration of the pure joy of the present moment can in large part be attributed to the Tantric Bhakti path, to the Tantric embrace of life in all its brutal and beautiful glory. Indeed, Shiva's Sanskrit aphorism, *Varttamanesu vartteta*, simply encourages us to *live in the present*. Shiva urges us to embrace life as it is, right now, in this very moment. Because, by living in the present, just like the Bauls of Bengal, our mind becomes intuitively receptive, fresh and open for spiritual revelation and rapture. Once, at a sacred Shiva festival in Nepal, I experienced yet more expressions of Tantric Bhakti Yoga in the form of the common people's devotion and adoration for Shiva. Each month of February, during the Shivaratri festival, hundreds of thousands of devoted pilgrims arrive at Pashupatinat temple from all over India and Nepal to honor the greatness of Lord Shiva. Preceding the pilgrims, and often the center of attention at the festival, half-naked *sadhus* arrive with matted hair and skin covered in ashes. Some sadhus can be seen demonstrating intricate yoga positions or sitting silently, lost in deep meditation. Others sit in lotus pose, explaining minute details of yogic philosophy. Long queues of devout Shiva worshipers snake up the temple steps, over the bridge and up the steps on the other bank. Devotees bathe in the shallow river and walk up the steps to enter the sacred temple, offerings in their hands. There I was in the middle of it all, a European dressed like an Indian yogi. I had come from far away to experience the ancient depths of Tantra for myself. I had come to dedicate my life to meditation, yoga exercises, vegetarian food, fasting, the singing of devotional songs, and the study of Sanskrit aphorisms and to serve humanity. Although a foreigner—a Viking among the indigenous followers of Shiva—I truly felt at home there.

The love for Shiva and the practice of Tantra are alive and well in India and the world today. Indeed, Shiva is undoubtedly one of the most popular deities in the Hindu pantheon. So, to claim that the Shiva devotees and ascetic yogis at Pashupatinat are not Tantric, as well as millions of others like them all over India, is to overlook the simple fact that India, in its cultural essence, is fused with the spirit and practice of Tantra. Danielou maintains that Hinduism owes much more to its pre-Vedic Tantric tradition than it does to the Vedic tradition. Bhattacharyya also observes that "Tantrism as a heterogeneous set of ideas and practices characterized the religious fabric of India—ancient, medieval, and even modern." And in the words of Anandamurtii: "Not only in India, but in quite a large part of the world, in every sphere of life, the laws and injunctions of Shiva alone prevailed for a long time. Even today the civilization of modern India is intrinsically Tantric. On the outside only is there a Vedic stamp." Furthermore, there is, in essence, no significant difference between Tantric Hinduism and Tantric Buddhism. As Anandamurtii reminds us, "Tantra is one and only one. It is based on one sentiment, on one idea."

And that one idea, that one spiritual destination, is achieved through Tantric practice, until one day our mind dissolves in Cosmic Consciousness, or Brahma. For the Tantric Hindu, this means to reach the lofty abode of *Parama Purusha*, and for the Tantric Buddhist, to be elevated to the state of *Shriman Mahasukha*. These are simply two different names for the same inward peaks of spiritual enlightenment.

The Aryan Controversy

In order to understand the ancient history of Tantra, one needs to understand the complex relationship between Tantra and the Vedas. Indeed, one needs to learn about the complex and often contentious relationship between the Vedic Aryans and the Tantric Dravidians of ancient India. So, let us venture on an exciting journey together, back in time to the beginning of humanity's ancient myths and spiritual teachings.

During my first journey throughout India, I discovered a country with great ethnic diversity. In southern India, I met Austric peoples whose facial features and complexion were similar to Africans or the Australian aborigines. In the south, east and west, I also met the generally tall and dark-brown complexioned Dravidians. In the north of India, and in Nepal, I met people whose facial features revealed various ethnic backgrounds. Some appeared Caucasian, some had light, yellowish skin and were Tibetan or Mongolian, and others had Dravidian features. It appeared as if I had arrived in an ethnic melting pot, a place where all the worlds' peoples had congregated. Indeed, India is composed of largely four main ethnic groups—the Mongolians, Dravidians, Austrics and Aryans. But where did these people originally come from?

It is not easy to piece together the vast tapestry of India's past. As mentioned earlier, most scholars thought for many years that Indian history started when ruthless, blue-eyed Aryans conquered the indigenous population in successive raids from 1900 BCE to 1200 BCE. Advocated by German-born Sanskrit scholar Max Muller, this theory made universal and bold claims. "The Aryan nations have become the rulers of history," he once wrote. In other words, Indian civilization was great only because of its white-skinned, Aryan origin. In Europe itself, the ideals of Aryan supremacy was, of course, promoted to its ultimate extreme by Adolf Hitler and his Nazi Party. Later in his career, though, Max

Muller retracted this idea. The Aryans, he ventured, indicated a group of people speaking Indo-European languages.

So what does the word Aryan actually mean? To the Vedic people in early India, the Sanskrit word *arya* meant "noble" or "cultured." In the ancient Vedic texts, the place between the Himalayas and the Vindhya Mountains were called *arya-varta,* or "the abode of the noble people." A third meaning is "the people from Iran." Aryan is also used by scholars as an ethnic or racial label for the Caucasian peoples. Then comes the next important piece of this historical puzzle: Since Max Muller advanced his invasion theory, there have been several alternative theories about the origin of the Aryan people in India. Most scholars now agree there was a succession of Aryan migrations into India, but they disagree about whether these ancients were warlike invaders or peaceful immigrants.

The idea that a group of noble, Vedic Aryans invaded a primitive Indian culture around 1500 BCE was overthrown in 1920 when the Indus Valley civilization was discovered. This discovery proved that the achievements of ancient India could no longer be credited to the descendants of the Aryan invaders alone. Why? Because the aboriginal Dravidians of the Indus Valley had planned cities and a standardized system of weights and bricks for at least two thousands years before the alleged invasion. Indeed, their civilization was more advanced than the nomadic tribes that supposedly conquered them.

But the controversy does not end here. Were the people of the Indus Valley Vedic, or were they Tantric? I had always taken for granted that they were Shaiva Tantric, because that is what I learned in India. But as mentioned earlier, a popular, alternative idea about Indian history today suggests the Aryan invasion theory is at worst based on a racist myth and at best on faulty scientific evidence. This idea has been promoted by some of the world's most prominent scholars on yoga, Tantra and Ayurveda. In other words, according to them, the Aryan invasion never happened. For these scholars, the only alternative appears to be that the Aryans must have been indigenous to India. In truth, they claim the Aryans are the "noble" and "cultured" people of Indian civilization, those who invented yoga, advanced spiritual philosophy, built the Indus Valley civilization and developed Ayurvedic medicine. But is this truly what happened?

As the word *arya* indicates, the Aryans could as well have been a people who came from outside India and settled in the Himalayas. Thus, according to Anandamurti, the pastoral, Caucasian nomads could at various times, have come to India through Iran from Central Asia. For the "new paradigm" scholars like David Frawley and Georg Feuerstein, however, there appears to be only one possibility: the Aryans have always been indigenous to India, and they are the people from the highest, noblest castes of society, most notably the Brahmins. For these authors, the Aryans represent all that is noble and great about Indian civilization, namely the Vedic cultural heritage. But is it true that the Aryans were simply noble and spiritual people?

The Real Story of the Vedic Aryans

The Vedas contain some of the most sublime philosophical truths humanity has ever conceived. Yet, the same Vedas, like all religious scriptures, also contain many dogmas and superstitions, including animal sacrificial rites to conciliate the gods. Moreover, the culture that advanced these texts also instituted a caste system in which millions of people to this day are treated as virtual slaves? In addition, surgery was forbidden by early Ayurvedic doctors due to possible "contamination" by lower castes. Women, according to many Vedic injunctions were considered too low to study and teach the scriptures. Indeed, it was only a few years ago a famous religious authority, the Shankaracharya of Sumerpeeth Kanchi, declared that women should not recite the *Vedas*. Such religious practices would be detrimental to their health and prevent them from having healthy babies, he claimed. Tantric teachings, on the other hand, have always been against the caste system and have generally held women in high regard. Indeed, it is inconceivable that an authority on Tantra would ever warn women from studying the scriptures. (Arvin, 1994)

So where did the Aryans come from? The idea of one single, violent invasion by barbarian Aryan hordes no longer seems plausible. This idea has been replaced by an immigration and acculturation taking place over a long period of time. Recent genetic and other scientific evidence supports this historical scenario. In fact, all the various peoples of India—the Austrics, the Dravidian, the Mongolians and the Aryans—came, at some point, from somewhere else. Indeed, all modern humans came from Africa.

Genetic and Linguistic Science and Ancient Indian History

On a rainy evening in 2003, I sat glued to the television screen watching the PBS program, *Journey of Man,* by Dr. Spencer Wells. The main reason I was so captivated by this program was that Dr. Wells offered scientific evidence for what Anandamurti and others had claimed—that the Aryan Vedic people migrated to India from Eastern Russia.

The genetic discoveries by Dr. Wells confirm the many stories I had heard from my guru, Anandamurtii, and from scholars and storytellers in India. Actually, his extensive research shows that India experienced four large migratory settlements over a period of nearly 55,000 years. By sampling DNA of people in a village close to Madurai in Tamil Nadu, he spotted a genetic mutation that had been passed on to aboriginal people in Australia—thus offering the first biological proof that African ancestors of the Australian natives passed through India on the way to their new home. His research also proved beyond a shadow of a doubt that the people who later moved into India in the north were of Aryan stock.

A few days after I had seen this captivating PBS program, I continued my research and located the interview (quoted in the introduction) with Dr. Wells in the online *Rediff* magazine. There he states emphatically that there is genetic evidence that "the Aryans came from outside India." The Rig-Vedic Aryan peoples, he claims, emerged on the southern steppes of Russia and the Ukraine about 5-8,000 years ago. From there, they migrated east and south through Central Asia toward India. Wells maintains that he is a scientist and does not want to take part in the religious debate about these issues. Thus saying, that he disagrees with scholars David Frawley and Georg Feuerstein, who claim the Vedic Aryans were the "original inhabitants" of India. To Wells, there is clear genetic evidence that "the Aryans came later, after the Dravidians."

A year later, I came across the research work of a team led by Michael Bamshad of the University of Utah in Salt Lake City. They compared the DNA of 265 Indian men of different castes with DNA from nearly 750 African, European, Asian and other Indian men. First, they analyzed mitochondrial DNA, which people inherit only from their mothers. When the researchers looked at specific sets of genes that tend to be inherited as a unit, they found that about 20 to 30 percent of the Indian sets resembled those in Europeans. The percentage was highest in upper-caste males, which is natural since the early Aryan settlers were by and large upper-caste Brahmins and Ksyattrias.

The genes that entered India when Aryan settlers emigrated from Central Asia and the Middle East are still there. And, according to these scientists from the University of Utah and from Andhra Pradesh University in India, they still remain entrenched at the top of the caste system. The invaders apparently subdued the local men, married many of their women and created the rigid caste system that exists even today. Their descendants are still the elite within Hindu society. Indeed, I had finally found scientific support for the stories I had heard from my Tantric guru in India.

Later, I learned from the work of geneticist Lynn Jorde of the University of Utah that "a group of males" was largely responsible for the Aryan invasion. If women had accompanied the invaders, the evidence should be seen in the mitochondrial genes, but it is not evident. The research team found clear evidence that women could be upwardly mobile, in terms of caste, if they married higher-caste men. In contrast, men generally did not move higher, because women rarely married men from lower castes. Since the caste system is still in vogue today, the same practice prevails.

Thus, as can be seen, genetic science corresponds with Anandamurtii's view that the Indo-Europeans, or true Aryans, indeed came from the outside and conquered the northern parts of the Indian subcontinent. The people they subdued—the Mongolians, Dravidians and the Austrics—descended from the original inhabitants who had arrived thousands of years earlier from Africa, the Middle East and other parts of Asia.

Finally, I pieced together information about the speakers of the various languages of India based, in part, on studies conducted by the People of India project of the Anthropological Survey of India. This project assigned the entire Indian population to 4,635 ethnic communities and putting together detailed information from over 25,000 individual informants from all over India. It was found that there are four major language families in India--Austric, Dravidian, Indo-European and Sino-Tibetan. These languages also correspond to the four main racial groups in India: the Austrics, Dravidians, Aryans and the Mongolians respectively. According to this study, it appears the Indo-European Aryans brought the Vedic language to India from Central Asia, a fact that has also been substantiated by the historical sequences and details outlined in Anandamurtii's many farseeing discourses on the history of India.

The main ethnic and linguistic groups that peopled ancient India.

Linguistic Group	Ethnicity	Arrival in India	Religion
Austric	Austric (Australoid)	60,000 BCE from Africa	Animism
Dravidian	Dravidian	10-8000 BCE from Near East	Proto-Tantra
Sino-Tibetan	Mongolian	10-8000 BCE from Far East	Proto-Tantra
Indo-European	Caucasian	6-4000 BCE from Central Asia	Rig-Veda

Unraveling the Genetic Controversy

It is often said that scientific facts are indisputable. Scientific data, however, are interpreted by human minds with often inadequate information and/or biased agendas. In the search for truth regarding India's past, fact is often confused with fiction and truth with biased opinions. One of the main reasons for that is that when we talk about history, we must also involve issues of culture, race and religion.

Questions about race and religion are often contentious and controversial. People's belief- systems run deep and strong, and so do people's opinions. In the past dozen years or so, I have often been attacked in online chat rooms, on Facebook and in articles for being "euro-centric, geo-centric, racist, chauvinistic and fascist." During one such heated debate, one of the participants, who supported my views, got so frightened by the violent rhetoric against us that he pulled out shortly after writing in a private email to me that he was "afraid for my family's safety." A couple of months later, however, to my great surprise and delight, one of the Indian antagonists wrote and apologized for his "shameful behavior and personal attacks" against us. Since then, his views have changed dramatically, and he is now openly supporting the Aryan migration theory.

So, what's all the controversy about? It is deeply rooted in the racial, cultural and religious history of India. However, India is not unique in harboring racism, sexism, bigotry and religious dogmatism—this is a human problem that exists in all countries, cultures and religions. Despite laws forbidding the caste system, issues of caste has become institutionalized in Indian culture and is often reflected in the debate about India's origins, including the issue about the Aryan migration theory, and most specifically regarding the issue of genetic science. Science is not always representing "the truth." Scientific conclusions are often reflections of the cultural and religious opinions of the interpreters of science.

In the December 2, 2005 Curriculum Commission hearing, supporters of the Vedic Foundation (VF) and the Hindu Education Foundation (HEF) in California, argued on the basis of a 1999 paper by the American genetic scientist Toomas Kivisild et al that the Aryan Invasion Theory had been "conclusively disproved" and should therefore be discarded from 6thgrade school textbooks. Based upon these arguments, the Curriculum Commission decided to accept various changes proposed by VF/HEF relating to the question of origin of the Aryans.

There is nothing controversial per se about these proposed changes. It is indeed common that new scientific facts often replace the findings of earlier scientists. But "new scientific facts" can also be colored or driven by political or religious opinions and agendas. It appears that this is the case in regards to the question of the Aryan origin debate.

The study by Kivisild et al focused primarily on the evolution/mutation of maternal genetic material (mitochondrial DNA) and did not take paternal genetic inheritance into account. The latter is important due to the fact that it was primarily men who first migrated into India and, most importantly, because men were less mobile in marriage in and out of caste than were women.

A 2001 study of male Y-DNA by both Indian and American scientists (including Toomas Kivisild) found that higher caste Indians are genetically closer to West Eurasians than individuals from lower castes. The genetic profiles of lower caste Indians, they discovered, are similar to other South Asians. These findings indicate that migrating male West Eurasians supplied a large genetic flow into the higher castes thus supporting the views asserted earlier, that the caste system was instituted by the predominantly male arrivals to keep themselves in a separate and dominating role toward the native population (Bamshad, 2001).

Both the genetic studies by Michael J. Bamshad and his team from the University of Utah and Dr. Spencer Wells' team give strong backing to the Aryan invasion/migration theory.In the study published by M.J Bamshad it is said that, "Our results demonstrate that for biparentally inherited autosomal markers, genetic distances between upper, middle, and lower castes are significantly correlated with rank; upper castes are more similar to Europeans than to Asians; and upper castes are significantly more similar to Europeans than are lower castes." (Bamshad, 2001)

Genetic studies shows that the Mitochondrial DNA is only passed on maternally, while the male-determining Y chromosome is passed along paternally. Thus the latter is used to study male inheritance. Despite religious and political protests from the fundamentalist Hindutva movement and its supporters, the genetic science consensus is that thousands of years ago Eastern European males invaded the Indian subcontinent and dramatically changed it forever.

Bamshad's scientific paper's abstract further states that, "In the most recent of these waves, Indo-European -speaking people from West Eurasia entered India from the Northwest and diffused throughout the subcontinent. They purportedly admixed with or displaced indigenous Dravidic-speaking populations. Subsequently they may have established the Hindu caste system and placed themselves primarily in castes of higher rank."(Bamshad, 2001)

The study also revealed another anthropological observation: that women have been significantly more mobile in terms of caste and hierarchical class than men. The latter are much less socially mobile in terms of caste and hierarchical class. Genetic evidence reveals how men have often married women from lower castes but that women have rarely been allowed to do the same with men.

In an online article published by Friends of Southeast Asia (FOSA), some of the most recent scientific studies are summarized as follows:

"In the 2003 study, Basu et al provide genomic evidencethat (1) there is an underlying unity of female lineages inIndia, indicating that the initial number of female settlersmay have been small; (2) the tribal and the caste populationsare highly differentiated; (3) the Austro-Asiatic tribals arethe earliest settlers in India, providing support to one anthropologicalhypothesis while refuting some others; (4) a major wave of humansentered India through the northeast; (5) the Tibeto-Burman tribalsshare considerable genetic commonalities with the Austro-Asiatictribals, supporting the hypothesis that they may have shareda common habitat in southern China, but the two groups of tribalscan be differentiated on the basis of Y-chromosomal haplotypes;(6) the Dravidian tribals were possibly widespread throughoutIndia before the arrival of the Indo-European-speaking nomads,but retreated to southern India to avoid dominance; (7) formationof populations by fission that resulted in founder and drifteffects have left their imprints on the genetic structures ofcontemporary populations; (8) the upper castes show closer geneticaffinities with Central Asian populations, although those ofsouthern India are more distant than those of northern India;(9) historical gene flow into India has contributed to a considerableobliteration of genetic histories of contemporary populationsso that there is at present no clear congruence of genetic andgeographical or sociocultural affinities."

Despite the scientific evidence to the contrary, there is often a political, religious, and ideological agenda behind the debunking of the Aryan migration theory and thus important aspects of the origins of yoga and Tantra. The proponents of this agenda have attempted to disprove that the Aryan people migrated from Eurasia towards India. Ironically, the Aryan migration debunkers call this a Eurocentric view, raised to prove that its proponents believe that everything great about India—namely its Vedic heritage—came from the outside, from people with greater wisdom and intelligence, and with lighter skin.

Here, I have attempted to establish quite the opposite view: that most, if not all, of the sophisticated ideas and practices related to yoga and Tantra, developed in India, but mostly *outside* the Vedic Aryan heritage, both before and after the Aryans crossed this continent's ancient and invisible borders thousands of years ago—by people with much darker skin. It is therefore rather unfortunate to witness how contemporary religious fundamentalism and political nationalism have come to dominate much of the writings and discussions about yoga's origins. Sometimes the views are overtly professed by propagandists, at other times covertly by the same group, and often unintentionally by undiscerning academics and practitioners. We have thus become witnesses to a retelling of the ancient past to fit a contemporary story that is both particular and universal: a whitewashing of important aspects of not only Indian history and the history of yoga, but also of the history of humanity itself.

The Vedic Aryans and the Tantric Dravidians—A Clash and Fusion of Civilizations

Sometimes when we study and practice Indian spirituality, Vedic and Tantric teachings will flow through us quite seamlessly, flow like a sacred river of spiritual wisdom. At other times, we will find the teachings to be distinctly different. Anandamurti often emphasized that the early parts of the Vedas, the Rig-Veda, were composed outside of India. This took place both long before and during the time of Shiva, at a time when these fair-skinned Aryan composers migrated into India.

Is there any proof of this? Authors like Bhattacharyya and Danielou have, for example, remarked on the lack of references to agriculture in the Rig-Veda. They think the main reason for this was that the early Aryans were pastoralists. In contrast, the Tantric Dravidians were rice-growing farmers. Moreover, you will not find any descriptions of the Indus Valley civilization in the Rig-Veda or even in the later Vedas. Nor will you find any references to the sophisticated grid pattern of streets. Nor will you find any mention of the careful engineering of the drainage systems, nor to granaries, warehouses and areas neither of intensive craft production, nor to the various seals found there.

Some Vedic scholars and writers on yoga argue that the Indus Civilization was purely a Vedic civilization. Popular writers like David Frawley, Georg Feuerstein, and Deepak Chopra promote this view. This so-called cradle of human civilization, they affirm, had few or no traces of Tantra. But is this a correct assertion? Marshall, Bhattacharya, Danielou, Chanda, and other scholars point out that the various artifacts found in these ancient ruins are, in fact, yogic or Tantric in nature. These include proto-Tantric fertility symbols such a lingams and yonis, or Mother Goddess figurines. The yogi Shiva, in the form of the Pashupati seal, is one of the most common figures found in these ruins. Here archaeologists have also discovered a marble statue of a yogi with eyes fixed on the tip of his nose. This marble statue displays a type of yogic gaze that I am quite familiar with. This trance-inducing gaze is actually an essential element in one of the Tantric meditation lessons I received many years ago. Thomas McEvilley points indeed out in his essay *An Archeology of Yoga* that this figure also represents a person engaged in some form of meditative practice. (McEvilley, 1981)

These archaeological finds, according to many scholars, all point in one direction— that Tantra was widely practiced in the Indus Valley civilization. This does not mean, however, that all members of this society were meditating yogis. Much like in today's India, we can assume that only a minority of the people were practicing Tantric meditation and yoga. Like today, most people were worshipers of various Gods and Goddesses, but not always practitioners of yoga's advanced spiritual sciences. Archaeological digs have also unearthed fire pits used for Vedic rituals in these old ruins. Therefore, I think it is reasonable to conclude that the Aryan and Dravidian peoples and cultures coexisted in northern India for several millennia. Indeed, by the time of the Indus Valley civilization, they probably lived together much like people from various castes, cultural and spiritual traditions coexist in India today.

This coexistence was not always peaceful. While the Rig-Veda contains hymns of sublime spiritual knowledge, including a few references to yoga, many of its stories are focused on the nature-worshiping rites of pastoral warrior clans. Some also tell colorful tales about the conquest of the "dark-skinned devils," namely the Dravidians of India. The Aryan priests made it painstakingly clear that non-Aryans (Anarya) were not allowed to pollute their culture and blood. In India you will find vestiges of this racist superiority even today. In personal ads in the newspapers, you will quite often find men and women looking for a marriage partner with "wheatish complexion." (Arvin, 1994)

So, what about all the symbolic references in the Vedas? Do all of them contain subtle messages of transcendental meaning? And do they therefore prove that the Vedas are the source of all Indian spirituality, including Tantra? When the Rig-Vedic people spoke of the Sun God Azura, for example, did they describe a deep state of meditation as some contemporary Vedic writers today want us to believe? Did they describe the "spiritual Sun within"? Since this was the age of magic and polytheistic power Gods, it is more likely that the early Vedic people thought the Sun had magical powers. (Wilber, 1996) Hence, they worshiped this bright, life-giving entity in the sky directly. They literally believed the sun was a God. In other words, to the early Aryans, the sun was not a symbol of a trans-rational state of meditation. Their devotion to the sun God Azura simply represented a pre-rational belief in the magical powers of that extraterrestrial and life-giving planet.

Indeed, most people at that time (12-6000 BCE) believed in a variety of nature's magical powers and spoke quite literally about those beliefs. Similarly, when the early Aryans called the dark-skinned people *devils*, they also meant it rather literally. They were not speaking of some symbolic struggle between good and evil. Their verses were often fearfully direct, and many symbolic references to higher, transcendental truths are often incorrect or were added later in the written versions. Anandamurtii pointed out that many of the Gods and Goddesses described in various Indian religious scriptures were, in fact, also representations of actual historical leaders. The Godman Krishna of Hindu mythology is a prime example, for he was, according to Anandamurtii, a non-Aryan Tantric yogi and a king who united Bharata (India) around 1500 BCE in a mighty war described in the classic epic *Mahabharata*.

Likewise, many of the mythological Gods of the Vedas, such as Indra, Agni and Varuna, were actual warrior leaders. Indeed, it was warrior leaders such as these who during thousands of years of gradual migrations and conquest finally conquered most of northern India. "It was not difficult for the healthy, martial, almost invincible Aryans to conquer northern India," writes Ananda-murtii. "The victorious Aryans treated the vanquished non-Aryans as slaves, trampling them underfoot to the bottom of their trivarna (three-caste) society—their society of Brahmans (priests), Ksyat-trias (soldiers) and Vaeshyas (merchants). There the non-Aryans became the fourth class, or Shudra Varna, while society became a caturvarna (four-caste) society." (Anandamurtii, 1984)

Thus, we can conclude that the so-called Indus Valley civilization eventually became a composite culture influenced by both Tantric and Vedic traditions. A similar merger between two civilizations took place in Europe when the Romans conquered Greece.

Harappa, Kashi and Mehrgarh—Ancient Cities of Tantra

While researching the complex history of India, I received help from many sources, from friends and books, from dreams and emails. One day, after I had a wonderful dream about Shiva, an email message from a friend, who had heard from another friend that I was writing a book on Tantra, alerted me to the connection between ancient Tantric peoples and the Tamil language of today.

The Tamil language of south India is considered one of the world's oldest living languages with its own script. An ancient Dravidian language, Tamil is more than 6,000 years old. In fact, an ancient form of Tamil, or Dravidian, is still spoken by the Brahui people today. These people's language and culture are indeed a living link back to the early dawn of Tantric history.

When the first Vedic Aryans migrated to India through the Khyber and the Bolan Passes, and mingled with the local population of the north, the north Indian proto-Dravidian languages changed to a great extent. However, in the area where the Brahui people still live, the old Dravidian language has remained virtually unchanged for millennia. The language of the Brahuis of Baluchistan, an area in Afghanistan and Pakistan, has many linguistic similarities to the Dravidian languages still spoken by the Tamils in south India today. Scholars have noted similarities in the numerals, personal pronouns, syntax and other linguistic features between Brahui and Tamil.

It is not only linguistics; however, that makes Baluchistan such an interesting historical area. This region, at the foot of the Bolan Pass, is also the site of Mehrgarh. Estimated to be more than 8,000 years old, it is regarded as the largest town of early antiquity. Covering an area of over 500 acres, Mehrgarh's population may have reached nearly 20,000 individuals. In comparison, the population of Egypt at the time was about 30,000. Living in brick houses, skilled in pottery making and the cultivation of rice, these ancient shamanic and proto-Tantric Dravidians were likely the first Indians encountered by the invading Aryans more than seven thousand years ago.

Urban culture was thus already in existence in India at the time of Shiva. Indeed, Mehrgarh had existed for almost two thousand years when Shiva was born. There is thus evidence of a continuous urban culture from Mehrgarh around 7000 BCE to the Harappan and Mohenjodaro civilizations in the Indus Valley around 4000 BCE. The current consensus is that the primary language represented by the Harappan script is related to modern Dravidian. The archaeologist Marshall was the first scientist to suggest a linguistic link between the Harappans and Dravidians.

As mentioned elsewhere, the complex and ancient Indus Valley civilization, which stretched from Afghanistan to the River Ganges, was largely a Tantra-oriented culture. In fact, the word "*hara*" refers to Shiva, and "*appa*" means father in the Dravidian language. The city of Harappa in the Indus Valley can thus be considered a place dedicated to Shiva, who by many today is considered the father of Indian civilization.

Since Tantra existed in India before Shiva, it is possible that the old Tantric civilization in India had its early roots in Mehrgarh, was systematized and refined during the time of Shiva, and continued to flourish for thousands of years in the Indus Valley civilizations of Harappa and Mohenjodaro. Most important, perhaps, Tantra remains alive and well in India and the rest of the world even today.

While Mehrgarh is the oldest archaeological city in the world, Kashi (today known as Varanasi) is the world's oldest living city. In Indian mythology, Kashi is considered the "original ground" where Lord Shiva and Parvati stood at the beginning of time. Benares is the point in which the first *jyotirlinga*, the fiery pillar of light by which Shiva manifested his supremacy over other Gods, broke through the earth's crust and flared toward the heavens. More significant than the cremation-ghats, and even the holy river Ganges, the Shivalinga in the Golden temple remains, to millions of Shiva devotees, the devotional focus of Kashi. (Wolfgang-Dieter, 2004)

Once again, Indian mythology leads us to a deeper understanding of history; the historical Shiva did, according to traditional sources, spend many years in Kashi, especially during the cool winter months, when Kashi, or Varanasi—the "holiest" city in all of India today—was his favorite resting place. Shiva's and Tantra's immeasurable contribution to humanity urges us to correct the common misconception that Tantra and yoga are relatively recent expressions of Indian spirituality. Indeed, the Classical Yoga period did not actually start with the famed *Yoga Sutras* of the sage Patanjali, but rather with Shiva, almost 5,000 years earlier. Most fundamental aspects of yoga—including many of the yoga exercises, breathing and meditation techniques used today—originated with the teachings of this great sage. What we today know as Hatha Yoga was consequently developed by Tantric sages over thousands of years, most notably expressed in writings by the Natha sect from 1000 CE onwards.

Irrespective of caste or creed, Tantra is a practical, timeless and visceral path, which over time reveals the innate spiritual intelligence of all those who embrace its philosophy and yogic practices. Hence, for many of those seeking spiritual emancipation through meditation and yoga in the West today, the historical Shiva, the King of Yogis, is re-emerging as a genuine archetype of yogic Enlightenment.

Brief history of Yoga and Tantra.

12000 BCE—Rigveda

The Rigveda was composed as an oral tradition outside India, but was not written down before 1700 BCE.

9-5000 BCE—Proto-Tantra.

Rudimentary forms of shamanistic Tantra practiced by Dravidians and Mongolians. Proto-Tantric city complex established at Mehrgarh around 7000 BCE.

5000 BCE—Tantra systematized by Shiva.

According to Shrii Shrii Anandamurti and others, Agama and Nigama, the philosophical and practical teachings, are given by Shiva and his wife Parvati. Shiva introduces the concept of Dharma—the path of spirituality and righteousness. He also introduces Tantra Yoga, including practices such as asanas, pranayama, dharana, pratyahara, and dhyana, as well as two versions of the Panchamakaras (Five Ms), one for the common people and one for yogis. Shiva also refines and systematizes Ayurvedic and Tantric medicine, often termed Vaedik Shastra. Moreover, Shiva formulates the marriage system, the musical octave and mudraic dances (with his wife Parvati). Tantra spreads to other parts of Asia, Europe and the Middle East.

5-2000 BCE—Tantra-oriented civilizations in India.

Tantric civilization established in Kota, Rajasthan, more than seven thousand years ago. Shiva establishes a city in Kashi (Varanasi), on the banks of the river Ganges. The Dravidians establish Tantra-oriented civilization in the Indus Valley region. People worship the Mother Goddess and also the Father God (Pashupati). Tantric yogis understand these expressions as Shakti and Shiva, the dual nature of Brahma.

5000-1500 BCE—Atharvaveda, Samaveda, Yajurveda

The three remaining Vedic texts were first composed orally in India by the Vedic Aryans after their arrival around 5000 BCE and then written as texts before or after 1500 BCE. Many Tantric passages are found in these texts, especially in the Atharvaveda.

2000 BCE—Transformation of the original Shiva Tantra.

Shiva Tantra (also termed the Shaivite tradition) transforms into two branches, the Gaodiya and the Kashmiri Schools. The Gaodiya

School was popular in East India (Bengal) and only marginally influenced by the Vedas.

1500 BCE—Krishna and Kapila

Krishna formulates three branches of yoga—action (Karma), devotion (Bhakti) and knowledge (Jnana). His teachings greatly influence the later school of Vaishnava Tantra. Yudhistira, a disciple of Krishna, popularizes the Tantric practice of pranayama, or breathing exercises. Tantric and yogic teachings spread all over the Far East. Maharishi Kapila formulates Samkhya, the world's first philosophy. Based on Tantra, the Samkhya philosophy is dualistic, but has many similarities to the non-dualistic Tantric philosophy to emerge some centuries later, forming the basis of Ayurvedic philosophy.

500 BCE—The Sramana Period

It is during this period scholars such as Mallinson and Singleton believe yoga started in the Sramana movement, but as indicated in this book, the Sramana movement was just another of many expressions of yoga which had its roots in Tantra at a much earlier date.

500 BCE—Gosala

During this period, Buddhism and Jainism was on the rise and Vedic society was beginning to decline. This was also the time of the Sramana movement, a yogic culture independent of Vedic hegemony. It was during this pivotal time in history, shortly before the arrival of the historical Buddha, that Gosala emerged as a Shaiva Tantric revivalist among various groups of yogis, such as the Ajivikas, the Kapalikas and the Kalamukhas. Gosala became the teacher of both the Buddha and Mahavira (the founder of the Jain religion) for several years.

400 BCE—Ashtavakra

This author of the well known nondual text The Ashtavakra Gita was also a famed Tantric who revived and popularized the Tantric system of Rajadhiraja Yoga, which was developed by Shiva thousands of years earlier.

200 BCE—Patanjali.

Inspired by both Tantra and Samkhya philosophy, Patanjali systematizes important aspects of Tantra into the eightfold path of Asthanga Yoga, which is basically his version of Tantric yoga. The Tantric idea that Brahma comprises both Shiva and Shakti was now widely accepted and consummated in the Ardha-Narishvara, an idol depicting half a man (Shiva) and half a woman (Shakti).

50 BCE—Lakulisha

Lakulisha re-awakens the old Shaiva tradition, or Tantra, during a time when both the Vedic culture and Buddhism was in decline. According to the Puranas as well as his own disciples, Lakulisha (the Club-bearing Lord) is considered to be the twenty-eight manifestation of Shiva. He restored the practices of Hatha Yoga, Tantrism and the cosmological ideas of Samkhya.

100 CE—Tirumular

Shiva Tantra adept from South India. A proponent of Bhakti Yoga and the author of the famed *Tirumantiram*, which is considered one of the greatest yogic canons of all time.

400-1200 CE—Tantra Shastras

Most of the important Tantric texts were written in this period, and thus to many scholars this was the "Tantric era" of Indian spirituality, but in reality the Tantric age started in 5000 BCE and lasted for thousands of years. Such texts include the *Kularnava Tantra* and the *Mahanirvana Tantra*.

600 CE—Age of Buddhist, Hindu and Jain Tantra begins.

Tantra Shastras are written and influence various schools of Buddhism, Hinduism and Jainism. Shiva Tantra evolves into five branches, or Paincha Tantra: 1. Shaeva Tantra, 2. Vaesnava Tantra, 3. Shakta Tantra, 4. Ganapatya Tantra, 5. Saura Tantra. Famous Buddhist Tantric yogis from this period and onward include Naropa, Milarepa, Saraha, Prahevajra, Je Tsong Khapa and Wanchuchuk Dorje.

800 CE—Yoga Vashista

This great Tantric yogi returns from China where he learned the subtle practice of Tantra meditation, which shows that Tantra came to China at an early age. His esoteric teachings on Tantric meditation and philosophy are compiled in the book, *Yoga Vashista*.

900 CE—Abhinava Gupta

This Tantric renaissance man revives Kashmir Shaivism, lays the foundation of Indian aesthetics, and writes an encyclopedia on nondualist Tantra.

1000 CE—Kularnava Tantra

This 17-chapter work contains over 2000 verses and even though it was influenced by Brahmanical thought, it is considered one of the most important Tantric texts.

1000-1200 CE—The Nathas Develop Hatha Yoga.

The founder of this movement, Matsyendranath, was a Shiva Tantric whose main disciple, Gorakshanath, systematized and further advanced the practices of Hatha Yoga.

1100 CE—Mahanirvana Tantra.

Considered by some as the most important of the Hindu Tantric scriptures, this fourteen- chapter text defines yoga in accordance with Shiva's teachings as the union of individual self (Jivatman) with the Cosmic Self (Paramatman).

1271-1296 CE—Jnaneshvar.

A genius Renaissance man and Tantric adept, Jnaneshvar composed the *Gitagovinda* at the age of 19, an epic poem reenacting the *Bhagavad-Gita*. Merging the Vaisnava movement with Kashmir Shiva Tantra, Jnaneshvar created a popular Bhakti movement in north India. The 19th-century sage Ramana Maharishi called him the "king of saints."

1300 BCE—Shiva Samhita

James Mallinson considers the Shiva Samhita a Tantric text dedicated to Lord Shiva from this period and not from the 17th century as most scholars believe. The text lists 84 different asana postures.

1500 CE—Hatha Yoga Pradipika

Written by Swami Svatmarama and dedicated to Lord Shiva, this text, together with Gheranda Samhita and Shiva Samhita, the three main surviving texts on Hatha Yoga linked to Matsyendranath and the Tantric Natha yogis. The book contains passages about pranayama, chakras, kundalini and various asanas and bhandas (locks).

1500 CE—Caetanya Mahaprabhu

A Tantric adept, Caetanya Mahaprabhu is undoubtedly the most well known and celebrated Bhakti yogis of India.

1500 CE-2000—CE Tantra Influences Many Spiritual Teachers and Paths

Some well-known spiritual teachers and leaders influenced by Tantra include Kabir, Guru Nanak, Paramahansa Ramakrishna, Swami Vivekananda, Swami Yogananda, Swami Shivananda, Swami Satyananda Sarasvati, Nityananda Avadhuta, Subhash Chandra Bose, Swami Laksman Joo, Swami Ram Thiirtha and Ramana Maharishi. Tantric philosophy and practices greatly influence several schools of Buddhism and, in general, all the movements within the Hindu yoga tradition. Contemporary Buddhist Tantric teachers include HH Dalai Lama, Lama Yeshe, Tulku Rgyen Rinpoche, and Jamyang Khyentse Chokyi Lodro.

1914 CE—John Woodroffe

The seminal book *The Principles of Tantra* is first published. Woodroffe's second classic on Tantra, *The Serpent Power*, was published in 1918.

1920s CE—Krishnamacharya

The modern yoga studio movement originated with T. K.V. Krishnamacharya and his school of yoga in Mysore, India. Krishnamacharya and his students claim that his practices are derived from an ancient text titled *Yoga Kuruntha*, but new research indicate that his system of asana practices are also combined with Western style gymnastics and poses of his own invention. Modern posture yoga practice as taught in today's yoga studios is a derivation of his style and those resulting from the innovations of his main students, B.K.S. Iyengar, Pattahbi Jois, Indra Devi, and his son T.K.V. Desikachar. Western students of these four trailblazers of modern yoga, including Rodney Yee, Richard Hittleman, Ganga White, and many more, have created numerous modified styles of their own, creating a booming multi-billion dollar yoga industry.

1921-1990 CE—Shrii Shrii Anandamurtii

Anandamurtii synthesizes the main features of Shiva's original teachings, incorporates Ashtanga Yoga, Hatha Yoga, unites the essence of the Five Schools of Tantra, and develop a comprehensive system of Tantra Yoga for the current era based on a new collection of Tantric sutras in the book *Ananda Sutram.*

Chapter Five
The Path of Union:
The Philosophy and Practice of
Tantric Yoga

THERE IS A MYSTICAL essence at the heart of all religions, which Aldous Huxley termed the "perennial philosophy." And there is perhaps no other spiritual path which epitomizes this essence more than Tantra. Indeed, some scholars believe that Tantra is the original religion, or the original spiritual practice, which lies at the heart of all mysticism and spiritual practice— whether in Islam, Hinduism, Buddhism, Jainism, Zen, and even mystical Christianity. In this last chapter of the book, we will take a deeper look at what Tantric philosophy and practice is all about.

Tantra: The Yoga of Sacredness

What is Tantric yoga? Most people in the West think of Tantra as a sexual practice. In India, however, most people think of Tantra as some kind of magical ritual performed by miracle working yogis. In reality, Tantra is neither. Tantra, like life itself, can be interpreted and experienced in a myriad of ways. As Tantric author Vimala McClure reminds us, Tantra is not the *yoga of sex nor magic*. Rather, she writes, Tantra is a holistic science and spiritual lifestyle we may term "the yoga of everything." (McClure, 1997)

As mentioned earlier in this book, there are various interpretations of what the word Tantra means. Some contemporary spiritual teachers explain that Tantra means *technique*. To them, the word connotes a transformative tool, a science, a way of life that brings joy and enlightenment. Some scholars says the word Tantra means *to expand,* as in expanding one's consciousness. Yet others will say that the word Tantra means *weaving.* Tantra thus signifies a kind of spiritual ecology expressed in concepts such as *nature's web of life* or the *interconnectedness of all that is.* Some religious scholars refer to Tantra as a cultural tradition that emerged in the early Common Era within Hinduism, Buddhism and Jainism. All these interpretations are partly right. Yet to truly understand the inherent spirit of Tantra, we must go to the root of the word and tradition itself.

As explained in previous chapters of this book, the Tantric tradition is thousands of years older than Hinduism, since the concept of Hinduism is only about 1000 years old. If we take a closer look at the Sanskrit scriptural definition of Tantra—tam jadyat tarayet yastu sah tantrah parikiirtiitah—then Tantra literally means that practice "which liberates a person from the bondage of inertia." (Anandamurtii, 1994)

The word Tantra, then, has two inner meanings: the path of *liberation from dullness* and the path of *personal expansion and enlightenment.* Moreover, a Tantric is someone who practices Tantra. Anandamurtii also writes that Tantra is a fundamental and universal spiritual science. Hence, Tantric practitioners can be found, irrespective of religion, wherever there is spiritual practice, wherever there is an attempt to attain spiritual liberation. In other words, even though Tantra as a specific path can be traced back to Shiva, in a more general sense, Tantra as the path of spiritual transformation is found among mystics of all religions, especially within Hinduism, Buddhism, Sufism, Jainism, Zen and to some extent within mystical Judaism and Christianity. In addition, Anandamurtii emphasizes that Tantra is both an internal and external path: "The Practice for raising *kulakundalini* is the internal sadhana of Tantra, while shattering the bondages of hatred, suspicion, fear, shyness, etc., by direct action is the external sadhana." (Anandamurtii,1979)

In its inner essence, Tantra is not a belief system, nor is it a religion. Tantra is a spiritual practice, a science and a philosophy that expresses the perennial source of the human quest for spiritual realization. As defined by the Bihar School of Yoga, Tantra is "the ancient science which uses specific techniques to expand and liberate the consciousness from its limitations." (Satyananda, 1984) Tantra thus represents our universal quest for truth within and beyond the world of material science and religion. Tantra is also a lifestyle. Based on a spiritual worldview and yogic practices, the Tantric lifestyle helps invoke the sacred in everyday life. In fact, the essence of Tantra—to quench our innate thirst for spiritual union—is at the heart of all yoga traditions. From Taoism to Hinduism, from Jainism to Buddhism, from medieval Kundalini yoga to contemporary Hatha Yoga, from traditional Raja Yoga to ecstatic Bhakti Yoga, the essence of Tantra flows as a seamless stream of transcendental knowledge. Because, in a more general sense, Tantra connotes the experiential and transformative mysticism at the heart of all the world's wisdom traditions. In that broad sense, both the Kali-worshiping Indian saint Ramakrishna and the God-intoxicated Christian mystic St. Theresa of Avilla were Tantrics. Their spirituality was not based on mere belief, but on spiritual practice, on their experience of union with the Divine.

Tantra, which often is termed Tantra Yoga, cannot be divorced from the inner essence of its own spiritual heart, from the experience of Bhakti, from the expression of spiritual love. American poet Robert Bly aptly describes Bhakti Yoga as the path where "the bee of the heart stays deep inside the flower, and cares for no other thing." (Bly, 1999) This focus on passionate love is integral to Tantra as it turns desire and attachment, the very antidotes of spiritual liberation, into an alchemical fuel for love and the emancipation of Spirit by worshiping all as God. Thus the bee of the heart goes so deep into what it loves that it transforms into love itself. To become that love is the goal of the love-intoxicated path of Tantra. This aspect of Tantra is especially expressed in

Vaishnava Tantra, where the love between Krishna and Radha epitomizes the spiritual union of Shakti and Shiva.

Tantric love is about creating spiritual oneness and union. Tantra is about feeling connected to the spiritual essence of the universe. And what is this essence? It has many names: God, Spirit, Godhood, Tao, Allah, or simply The One. In Tantric cosmology and philosophy, this essence is called Brahma, or Cosmic Consciousness. And this Brahma is composed of pure Cosmic Consciousness, or Purusha (Shiva) and pure energy, or Prakrti (Shakti), the dual expressions of Brahma. Just like light and heat are inseparably one with fire, Shiva and Shakti are the inseparable yet dual expressions of Brahma.

Shiva is Brahma as pure Cosmic Consciousness, and Shakti is Brahma as Cosmic Creative Energy, the force behind creation, the force that created you and me, the plants, the animals and the earth. Shiva and Shakti, like a wave and a particle in quantum physics, are never separate. They are always together, always the same. They are simply two different expressions of the same universal Brahma. Remembering these primal aspects of the world, we open up to see and experience oneness in duality everywhere. We open up to feelings of spiritual connectedness and love.

The primal, evolutionary force of Shakti—which is both real and symbolic—is that which inspires us toward illumination and wisdom. Yet the same force has the capacity to blind us, to drive us away from truth and self-realization. In other words, the duality of wisdom and ignorance, Vidya and Avidya Shakti, exists at the very root of creation and life itself. Thus, no matter at which stage we are on the spiritual path, there is always the possibility of making mistakes. Hence, there is always a need for spiritual vigilance, always a need to personify a deep, spiritual ethic, and always a need to embrace and transcend our own limitations and ignorance.

Our challenge is to go beyond the illusion of Avidya Shakti. When we take up that challenge, we are inspired to reach our natural state of spiritual being. And when we live and breathe from that state, we are supported by the spiritual power of Vidya Shakti. We will experience more and more synchronicity, harmony and vitality in our life. Still, after the spiritual light has awakened us, we must be vigilant. Tantra is thus a dynamic path and urges us to stay awake in the light of spiritual being at all times.

The path of Tantra is about experiencing spiritual bliss, to soak the human heart with divine Spirit. Thus, it is often said that Bhakti Yoga, the path of ecstatic love, is the best and safest path. This Yoga of Love is beautifully exemplified in the life and poetry of Rumi, who said, "The taste of milk and honey is not it. Love instead that which gave deliciousness." In other words, love that which is within and beyond all physical forms and expressions. Love that which is within and beyond food, sex, fame, and money. As the Tantrics will say, when you cultivate love for that which gives you all that is delicious in life, namely Brahma, you will eventually experience love in everything. That is the spirit of Tantra. That is the alchemy of Tantric love.

This, then, is the path of Vidya Tantra—the path that leads us to experience the unity of Shiva and Shakti in our own hearts and minds, and, hence, to the realization of Cosmic Consciousness everywhere.

Tantra Is Yoga, and Yoga Is Tantra

If you are one of the millions of people today who practice yoga at home or in a studio, you are practicing a form of Tantra. Because, just as the world of Tantra is often viewed through a narrow lens today, so is the case with yoga. Some enthusiastic practitioners of these exercises endure 105-degree sweats at a Bikram Yoga studio in downtown smoggy Los Angeles. Others start their day with a sun salutation exercise at a pristine yoga retreat in Hawaii. Yet others find it more convenient to practice at home watching their favorite yoga teacher on DVD. No matter which style, these yoga postures, or asana, which literally means "comfortably held positions," enhance physical well-being. But physical health was not the only reason Tantric yogis developed these exercises.

Traditionally there are actually two categories of these exercises: one is primarily for physical health and secondarily for spiritual growth, and one is primarily for concentration and spiritual growth. The well-known *padmasana,* or Lotus Pose, belongs to this second category. Originally, asanas were prescribed to better prepare us for the spiritual aspects of yoga, namely the practice of long and deep meditation. With these insights in mind, we can now better understand why the Tantra yogis termed the body a physical temple of the Divine Spirit.

The promises of health, relaxation, longevity and spiritual enlightenment have inspired many to take up the ancient practice of yoga today. Common to all modern yogis is the practice of some aspect or version of Hatha Yoga. Not all yoga students are aware, however, that their practices—whether it is asanas practiced as Bikram Yoga, Iyengar, Power Yoga, Kripalu or Kundalini Yoga—have deep roots in the teachings of the medieval Tantric sages Matsyendranath and Gorakshanath.

The achievements of this miracle worker and saint from the ninth century CE build on the tradition laid down in earlier eras by Tantric yogis, including Matsyendranath, the founder of the Shiva-oriented Natha sect. The practice of Hatha Yoga culminated in the writing of the Hatha Yoga Pradipika text around 1500 CE. Both the teachings of Gorakshanath and those in the Hatha Yoga Pradipika emphasize the importance of blending Hatha Yoga with Raja Yoga, which is just another way of saying that Hatha Yoga is best combined with Tantra, since Raja Yoga, according to Anandamurtii and others, originated in the Tantric teachings taught by Shiva thousands of years earlier.

Tantra: The Yoga of Union

The term Tantra basically means *the path of liberation,* but what does the Sanskrit word yoga mean? Here again, there are various interpretations. The two most important are offered by Patanjali and by Shiva. Patanjali explained in his famed Yoga Sutras that yoga means *the suspension of all mental tendencies or propensities.* In other words, one attains inner peace when the mind is void of distractions, void of thought and feelings. This rather dry definition of yoga never quite took hold in Indian culture. Shiva's popular Tantric definition is more heart-centered and soulful and has come to signify the most popular definition of yoga, not only in India but all over the world. Yoga, said Shiva, is that *process which creates union between the individual soul (jivatman) and the Cosmic Soul (paramatman), yoga is that which creates union between Shakti and Shiva.* (Anandamurtii, 1994)

In plain English, yoga is also the inner state of wellbeing we feel when there is harmonious interaction between body, mind and spirit. As a lifestyle, yoga is a path of self-discovery. Through asanas and meditation, yoga promotes physical health, mental balance and spiritual peace. Spiritually, yoga means *union* and refers to the state of enlightenment. As an art and a science, yoga aids us in developing a more healthy and balanced lifestyle.

The spiritual state of yoga, or union, is often expressed through spiritual love or Bhakti Yoga. In traditional temple sculptures, the unity of Shiva and Shakti, as well as our spiritual, nondual union with the Divine, is symbolized by two lovers in a tight embrace. In the Mayatantra, one of the ancient texts based on Shiva's teachings, yoga is similarly defined as "the unity between the individual soul and the universal soul." In the Kularnavatantra, the attainment of yogic union is poetically described as "water pouring into water." Hence, Tantra and yoga are like Shiva and Shakti, like two sides of one single sheet of paper. You cannot really have one without the other.

The Many Faces of Tantra

The spirit of Tantra implies a dynamic effort to overcome the dominance of Avidyamaya, the forces of ignorance and lethargy that keep us away from doing the inner work needed to attain enlightenment. These dynamic, physical, mental and spiritual efforts can be carried out in largely three ways and are characteristic of the three main paths of Tantra.

The Right-hand Path. Termed Dakshina Marga Tantra in Sanskrit, this so-called Right-hand Path attempts to overcome Avidyamaya, or ignorance and darkness, through the use of idols, devotional chanting and prayer to the Gods and Goddesses. It is imperative on this path of Bhakti Yoga to realize that the symbolic representations of the Divine are just gateways to the Spirit realm. They are internal archetypes of the mind and Spirit. Religious people with a pre-rational mentality often interpret their symbols and ideas literally. This is a potential limitation with such worship. It can lead to religious literalism and, even worse, to fundamentalism and dogmatism. People on this path also tend to pray to receive boons from God, rather than to praise the Divine with chants, music and poetry in order to feel oneness with God. So, in order to harness the spiritual potential of this path most effectively, one must also understand these potential trappings. Yet even for those of a rational or even transrational (mystical) state of mind, such as the great sage Ramakrishna, there are subtle aspects of this popular path to consider. Ramakrishna, who was famous for his worship of Mother Kali, or Shakti, and who worshiped Her as a gateway to the realm of pure Consciousness, achieved high states of spiritual enlightenment, but not the most sublime state of *nirvikalpa samadhi*, or complete enlightenment.

It was only when the naked wanderer and Tantric guru Totapuri initiated him in the practice of nondual mantra meditation that Ramakrishna attained oneness with Cosmic Consciousness. He did so after Totapuri pressed a piece of glass into his forehead and told him to concentrate his mind in that point. Then, by piercing through the dualistic veil of Goddess Kali, Ramakrishna attained *nirvikalpa samadhi*, or nirvana. He remained in this mystical trance for three days continuously, a state that Totapuri himself had taken many years to attain. After that seminal experience, Ramakrishna was able to move in and out of this exalted world of nondual bliss with effortless grace for the rest of his life.

The Left-hand Path. Termed Vama Marga Tantra in Sanskrit, this path attempts to overcome the deceptions of Avidyamaya by "any means possible" but sometimes without a clear goal of attaining yoga, or spiritual union. This path is legendary for its highly advanced sexual practices and the explicit use of occult powers. Hence, it is also often considered a path of Avidya Tantra, or the kind of black magic that Tantra is famous for in India. The main challenges on this path are the many temptations for misusing one's physical and psychic desires and powers.

Some Tantric adepts on this path claim they have transcended all worldly attachments while making a show of doing whatever they wish—they drink heavily; they have excessive sex with multiple partners; they live in riches. While it is possible, through intense inner discipline, for yogis to become enlightened through left-handed practices, it is nevertheless a risky path. Fraught with many contradictions and dangers—both for student and teacher—this path has many pitfalls and often lacks any clear ethical or cultural customs to be guided by.

In some schools of Left-hand Tantra, however, a disciple will follow strict codes of discipline and morality until he or she is allegedly enlightened and ready to lead the unconventional life of a Crazy Wisdom teacher. Because the Left-handed Path appeals to our contemporary excesses of sex, ego, fame and entertainment, it is often this path's sexual excesses that are labeled Tantra in the West. In reality, this sexual path is quintessentially not representative of traditional Tantra.

The Middle Path. Termed Madhya Marga Tantra in Sanskrit, this so-called Middle Path is what is mainly taught by the traditional gurus of Tantra, and it is the most common school of Tantra Yoga. While all three of these paths originated with Shiva, this is the path he prescribed for those who want to immerse themselves in the path of spiritual yoga practices. This path has been further advanced throughout the ages by various gurus and adepts, including one of the most revered sages of the past century, namely Anandamurtii. It is generally considered the most mindful and dependable path. This *middle path* toward realizing the spiritual effulgence of Brahma removes Avidyamaya's veil of ignorance through an integrated and balanced set of physical, mental and spiritual practices. Some also refer to this as The Direct Path since it employs mantras and visualization techniques to focus the mind to go beyond the mind and into a state of pure, flowing meditation.

Tantric sages advise us to inquire into our own deepest self, into our own state of pure being by transcending the analytical and feeling mind and its false sense of egoic self. But to achieve this state of pure Being is not as easy as it sounds. It is much easier to think that you have achieved pure Being, to have an intellectual idea of what that means, than actually to be in a state of pure Being. The Tantric Middle Path prescribes a radical yet indirect way to gradually achieve a transcendental state of being: simply by focusing the mind through meditation on the breath with a mantra, which is literally a tool *to liberate the mind*. While using the breath and a mantra to still and focus the mind's chatterbox, you gradually transcend the mind itself. To use the mind to transcend the mind, a seemingly contradictory practice, represents the real essence of Tantric transformation. Breathing exercises, or pranayama, is another practice that aids in the process of accessing the deep waters of spiritual illumination, as pranayama makes it much easier to concentrate and thus to still the mind. In addition, Tantric meditation also employs chakra and yantra visualizations as well as devotional chanting and dancing.

Dr. Chris Kang, a Tantric practitioner who holds a doctorate in Religion, has written extensively on Tantra and Buddhism. Once, during an e-mail exchange we had about Tantra, he emphasized yet another equally crucial element in Tantric meditation: to use the meaning of the mantra to direct the mind's attention toward its own nature. That is, we are not simply focusing or stilling the mind in one-pointed awareness, but also clarifying and sharpening our awareness so that it sees and knows directly the ultimate nature of the mind itself. This type of insight is possible because the mantra's meaning activates the mind's innate reflexivity and catapults the conceptual mind beyond itself and into its underlying, blissful luminosity. Hence, our awareness sees and knows itself by becoming itself in its natural state.

Mantra, chakra and breath meditation facilitates this process, which begins with deep breathing, or *pranayama*, intense sensory withdrawal, or *pratyahara*, in combination with focus on a chakra and a mantra, or *dharana*, and ends in inner flow meditation, or *dhyana*, and then finally union with the deep inner Self, or *Samadhi*. This practice, which is essentially Tantric sadhana, or meditation, is the process of the mind accessing its own spiritual luminosity.

In addition to these three paths, there are broadly five different schools of Tantra that developed during the early Middle Ages, thousands of years after Shiva developed the essential yoga and meditation practices still in use today. These are the Shakta, Vaesnava, Shaiva, Ganapatya and Saura Tantra schools. Moreover, when Jainism and Buddhism flourished in India, various branches of Buddhist and Jain Tantra, developed, which again sprouted many independent branches. The early Middle Ages also spawned such fabled paths as the Left-handed Aghora Tantra—today popularized in the West by the books of Robert Svobodha—as well as the well-known Buddhist Vajrayana Tantra. By this time, many Tantric schools had synthesized with the Vedic tradition, and Shiva Tantra lost some of its original form until it again was revived by Anandamurtii during the last century.

Tantra and Sex

Tantra is often associated with sacred sex. In Western neo-Tantra, this is the main focus. But that is not what traditional Tantra is all about. The common misconception in Western New Age circles, that sexual Tantra is some kind of pathway toward salvation, is contrary to the inner essence of this ancient and sublime practice. Because true, lasting pleasure comes, according to Tantra, not from physical objects and attachments, but from within.

The left-handed path of Tantra was originally prescribed by Shiva as a path of moderation, not excess, as is often the case at seminars promoting what is commonly termed Neo-Tantra and some humorously refer to as Hot Tub Tantra, or California Tantra.

The main idea behind the original practice of the left-handed path is to practice spirituality (sadhana) while in the midst of enjoyments. This path was, according to Anandamurtii, also prescribed by Shiva, as a means of reducing one's intake of wine and meat and, at the same time, to harbor spiritual feelings while relishing their delights, and ultimately to rise above the transient nature of these earthly pleasures all together.

For the spiritually inclined yogis, those who want more than material wealth and physical pleasures, the Five M's have a different, more subtle meaning. As Georg Feuerstein writes, "[in some] schools [the Five M's] are understood symbolically and are completely internalized." (Feuerstein, 1998)

Here, based on the teachings of Anandamurtii, is a brief overview of these ancient Tantric aphorisms and how to interpret the Five Ms when they are internalized:

Madhya (wine)–to enjoy the *sudha* or *somadhara*, which, while in deep meditation, is a hormonal secretion from the pineal gland. A second meaning is that it refers to the spiritual aspirant's ecstatic or intoxicated love of God.

Mamsa (meat)–one who has control over his or her speech, or one who surrenders all actions–good, bad, sinful, righteous, or wicked–to God, is said to be a practitioner of *mamsa* yoga.

Matsya (fish)–refers to the subtle science of pranayama (breathing exercises), and also to the feeling of deep compassion arising in a spiritual person's heart.Mudra (grain)–avoidance of bad company, as bad company leads to bondage and good company leads to liberation.

Maethuna (intercourse)–the purpose of maithuna yoga is to raise the Shakti (divine energy, also called kundalini), located at the lowest vertebrae of the spine, and unite it with Shiva in the spiritual energy center at the top of the head, the *sahasrara* chakra.

So while Tantra has nothing against sex, it is also not a path focused exclusively on sacred sex, which is often the impression given by practitioners of Western neo-Tantra. The main traditional school of Tantra in which sexual magic is a key element is the path of Kaula Tantra. But Tantra as developed by Shiva is best described as a comprehensive spiritual science, which is what the word Tantra itself implies—a path of transformation, a path to inner liberation. Thus Tantra is the spiritual science that liberates the spiritual practitioner or yogi from limitations, from the mind trapped in delusions, be they physical, mental or spiritual. Tantra is thus a path, not about sexual indulgence, but a path that personifies the very essence of yogic nondualism, of seeking the ultimate and infinite pleasure: oneness, or union with the Divine.

Is Tantric Yoga a Religion or an Intuitional Science?

The word religion comes from the Latin *religare*, which means to unite again with the Source, or with God. In other words, the word religion means much the same as the word *yoga*, which in its Tantric definition means *"to unite, to become one with."*

Throughout history saints from various religions have described their ecstatic experience of God-intoxication as gnosis, *samadhi* or *satori*. Religion in its truest sense is thus a path, which, if practiced diligently, eventually leads to the experience of unity with God, Spirit, Allah. In its truest, deepest essence, religion is yoga, the practice of spirituality.

But that's not always the case. Religion has also been one of the most divisive and bloody forces on the planet—the source of many despicable dogmas and irrational creeds we can sure live without. In some Vedic scriptures, such as in the Vedic Book of Manu, we will find many such dogmas and irrational tenets—against women or outcasts—which have little to do with the inner spirit of yoga or Tantra. Similarly, in some so-called Tantric schools one may also find practices that are also riddled with dogmas or superstitions.

As stated earlier, the ancient Tantric concept of yoga means to become "one with *paramatman*, one with the Cosmic Soul." Yoga, in other words, is the state of mind when our individual soul experiences oneness with the Cosmic Soul, or with God. Thus, at the mystic heart of every religion lies an understanding that there is an all-pervasive state of reality–God, Brahma, Tao—and that this reality can be experienced within through the practice of yoga, meditation, prayer, or chanting.

"The Kingdom of God is within you." (Luke 17.21)

As comparative religious scholar Huston Smith has explained, each religion embraces the Great Chain of Being. According to this view, humans throughout history have viewed reality as a hierarchy of levels–from matter to body to mind to spirit. All these levels are ultimately enfolded by the Source, the Ground of Being, by God, Consciousness, or Spirit.

But unfortunately religion is not always the same as spirituality. Religion has often kept people away from the experience of spirituality.

"Thou shall have no other gods before me." (Ten Commandments)

"A widow should be long suffering until death, self-restrained and chaste. A virtuous wife who remains chaste when her husband has died goes to heaven. A woman who is unfaithful to her husband is

reborn in the womb of a jackal." (The Laws of Manu, Chapter 5 verse 156-161, Dharmashastras, a sacred Hindu text)

While the originators of the great religions may have experienced a deep sense of union with Universal Consciousness and also subscribed to the near universal belief in the Great Chain of Being. The same religions, which generally were established years after the founders died, or during times when cruel practices such as widow burning or sacrificial killings of animals and humans were commonplace, are thus often riddled with myths and dogmas. That is, religions are often the opposite of spirituality.

The Hindu Vedas, for example, contain some of humanity's most ancient and sublime spiritual revelations, but Hinduism has also adopted many dogmatic injunctions (such as the caste system) that serve to separate and discriminate rather than unite and embrace people. Hinduism, like all religions, contains many irrational myths: a dip in the sacred Ganges in the holy city of Varanasi (Benares) will bring you to heaven when you die; only men from the Brahmin caste can be priests. There are also many fundamentalist followers of Christianity who believe in such irrational ideas as the virgin birth, the physical resurrection, and that creation was consummated in only six days.

No wonder the exponents of science and rationality revolted against such illogical doctrines. But scientific rationalism has also failed miserably in its critique of the innermost spiritual truths of religion, in its critique of what is often called "perennial philosophy," "universal truths," or simply "spirituality." Because objective science and rationality cannot describe, experience or proclaim the truth or veracity of something that can only be experienced subjectively and is beyond the rational. Objective science can determine that you meditate, but the same science cannot describe your spiritual experience. Even the person experiencing samadhi will have an impossible task explaining how it feels.

The rational can only approximate the trans-rational. Objective science can never fully explain subjective truth. That is why even scientists resort to poetry, to myth, to explain certain objective truths. That is why we have language, why we have maps. But language and maps are not the same as reality, neither objective nor subjective realty.

Ilya Prigogine is best known for his definition of dissipative structures and their role in thermodynamic systems far from equilibrium, a discovery that won him the Nobel Prize in Chemistry in 1977. He likened his discovery, which basically reverses the second law of thermodynamics, to the dance of Shiva. Because in closed thermodynamic systems there is no exchange of energy or entropy with the environment. There is dynamic equilibrium. Thus his evocation of Shiva's dance, who dances in eternal dynamicity beyond both life and death.

So, both science and religion uses metaphor to explain certain truths. The problem arises when we take the metaphors—the virgin birth, the resurrection, the virgins in heaven, the flames of hell, the matter-is all-there-is, the-brain-is-all-there-is theories—literally. That's when the trouble starts. Trouble starts when we take all that science has to offer and believe that is all there is. No wonder we have ended up with a world of lean yogis without soul, buildings without sacredness, things without depth.

There's trouble when science says that the sensory world is everything. Objectivity is everything. We end up with a flat world devoid of inner transcendence, inner subjectivity, inner spirit. But those scientists who understand the mystery, the sacred, they become poets, mystics, spiritualists. Why? There is simply no other way to explain the unexplainable.

As Albert Einstein said, *"The most beautiful and most profound experience is the sensation of the mystical. It is the source of all true science."*

Benedictine monk and author David Steindl-Rast explains the importance of distinguishing between the essence of religion and its institution or dogmas: "Religion...should be written with a capital R to distinguish it from the various religions. Translated into everyday living, Religion becomes spirituality; institutionalized it becomes a religion." (Steindl-Rast, 1992)

The main point here is not one of semantics but to understand the essence of what some call Religion, universal religion, the perennial philosophy, or simply spirituality. Or dharma. Which is the same as spirituality and Religion, but very different from religion with a small r.

The Sanskrit word *dharma* means "an object's or a being's inner nature." In the context of humanity's search for perennial wisdom, spirituality is the dharma or inner characteristic of that human condition. In fact, dharma is often translated as "the spiritual path." Dharma just is, and to be human is to become one with that which just is.

Thus spirituality supports and includes rationality and science. Religion, in its various guises, on the other hand, is often based on a literal translation of irrational myths and legends and thus is often in conflict with both human nature and science. Thus we cannot equate Hindu Dharma, or any other religious creed, as human dharma, as universal dharma.

Because religions generally depend more on scripture and belief rather than, as in spirituality, on practice and experience, we may term it a dogma. It is also often in conflict with basic human values and therefore unable to inspire and guide humanity on its march toward creating a universal and truly integrated society. So, for the sake of a theoretical definition of the difference between religion (dogma) and spirituality (dharma), let us say that religion contains both certain universally accepted truths as well as many irrational dogmas, while spirituality soars beyond and above these irrational limitations. It contains truth, beyond words, truth that can only be approximated by poetry, dance, song, truth in its most unblemished and sacred form.

Another way of making this distinction is to say that religion, with its emphasis on external rituals, is exoteric, and that spirituality, with its emphasis on sacred, meditative practice, is esoteric. In conclusion, spirituality, not religion, is the only power that is universal, sublime, and silent enough to truly unite human society. This is essence has been the inner message of yoga throughout the ages.

Yoga and Activism

"A mysticism that is only private and self-absorbed leaves the evils of the world intact and does little to halt the suicidal juggernaut of history; an activism that is not purified by profound spiritual and psychological self-awareness and rooted in divine truth, wisdom, and compassion will only perpetuate the problem it is trying to solve, whatever it's righteous intentions." –Andrew Harvey

Enlightenment, in other words, is not an escape from the world but a true return to the world. In the words of sages and pundits from various wisdom traditions and backgrounds, we see a common, golden thread: enlightenment is being in this world but not of it. Enlightenment is having your head and heart in the wide open sky of spirit and your feet firmly planted in the garden of life.

In other words, enlightenment means transformation, transforming us and the world at the same time. Enlightenment means to be an integral person working toward creating an integral world. Enlightenment means being a spiritual activist. So what do the great wisdom traditions say that urges us to be active in this world? From Buddhist and Hindu Tantra, we learn:

"Brahma (Cosmic Consciousness) is the world."

"Nirvana and samsara are not two."

"Shiva (Cosmic Consciousness) and Shakti (Cosmic Energy) are one."

"Brahma is the composite of Shiva and Shakti."

In other words, the nondual philosophies of Tantric Yoga, for example, teaches us about inner and outer ecology; that the world of spirit (Shiva) and the world of matter (Shakti) are essentially an integrated whole; are one in Brahma.

In the words of Ken Wilber: "The point, we might say, is that the circle of Ascending and Descending energies must always be unbroken: 'this world' and the 'other world' united in one ongoing, everlasting, exuberant embrace." (Wilber, 1996)

In the words of Tantric guru, Anandamurtii: "Yoga means unification…We must have yoga in all the three levels of life. If there is yoga only in the spiritual level and there is no yoga in the psychic and physical level, what will happen? The very existence of human beings will become unbalanced, human equipoise will be lost. So we must have yoga, or rather yoga-oriented movement, in each and every sphere of life." (Anandamurtii, 1984)

But not all yoga philosophies have urged the same balance; not all yogis have lived firmly rooted in this world. In Vedanta we are taught that this world is an illusion. Consequently some yogis have fled this world to seek salvation in spirit only. There are always exceptions. Even though Vivekananda was a follower of Vedanta and did not think posture yoga (asanas) was very important, he was a political activist in his native India.

So, what does it mean to practice "Yoga in each and every sphere of life?" It can simply mean that when we buy yogurt, we consider not only how deliciously it melts on the tongue and how good it is for health but also how good it is for the planet's health—we will also consider how and where the yogurt was produced. That is one simple to practice yoga in every sphere of life, that one way to practice yogic ecology. If all is one, the way our food is made and where it comes from matters. If all is one, the less suffering I cause animals and the environment matters. If all is one, as yoga says, it all matters. Not just my personal body and soul, but also the body and soul of others, the body and soul of animals, of plants.

To be a yogi activist, then, is to look the world straight in its face and answer all the uneasy questions in life and come up with workable, conscious compromises. Because, here on this dusty earth, perfection, like the sexy perfection in that sleek, sensual body of the Lululemon yogi, that kind of perfection is not the perfection the yogi activist will always find or even want.

Yogi perfection is, first of all, a state of mind, a state of heart, a state of consciousness; then that state of mind urges us into imperfect action. Imperfect action in the world of Shakti, the world of samsara.

Still, we act by thinking, by feeling, that this world is also Brahma, also Consciousness, also sacred. In Tantra that is acting from the state of *madhuvidya*, from the heart of honey knowledge. We act as if the world is a sweet and sacred place to live. Always.

That which is broken can heal, and that act of healing is yoga, that act of healing is spiritual activism. That act is part of the idea that samsara and nirvana are one, the idea that Shiva and Shakti are one in Brahma. The idea of the European Alchemists who said that "what is above is also below."

That is Tantra, that is yoga. That is what the yogic transformation enterprise is all about: to blend that which is within us with that which is outside us. That is the sacred and often complex and neglected enterprise of yoga.

Yoga can mend ligaments, backs, hearts—and yoga can, in small and big ways, mend the world.

According to Anandamurtii's Tantric interpretation of yoga, the path of yoga combines self-realization and service to the world. Because, if yoga is all about navel gazing and retreating from this world, then what kind of yoga is it? The yoga of a selfish, lonely, separated soul in the body of a sexy Lululemon ad? The yoga of a body-denying ascetic whose nails are too long to feed himself?

It is no accident that religious enterprises which are about going-to-heaven-only and yogic enterprises which are for-myself-only have a one-dimensional resemblance to economists who define human behavior and aspirations in purely economic terms. The economic human sees greed as good; that selfish aspirations are solely what an economy is built upon. And that fictionalized version of reality has created a fictionalized, phantom economy based on greed and speculation.

Likewise, the ego-driven yogi mistakes the beautiful body in the mirror for the beautiful self within. And the ascetic thinks that by denying the body it will eventually evaporate into the transparent purity of soul. Body obsession and profit obsession and ascetic-escaping-the-world obsession thus share similar traits: they have great difficulty embracing reality in its wholeness, in its imperfect, complex yet sacred earthiness.

If yoga is holistic, which I believe it is, then part of its holism lies in its ability to embrace opposites and see the oneness in diversity and complexity. Yoga thus is not only about occupying the mat, the cushion and Wall Street, but about occupying the whole of reality, the whole of life in all its divine, imperfect and vast sacredness—in each and every moment of our lives. That, and nothing less, is the yoga of imperfect perfection, the yoga of enlightenment with both a small and capital E. That is the Tantric yoga of sacred activism.

The Tantra of Inner Transformation

Some people on the spiritual path claim that we do not need to transform, do not need to change in order to be spiritual. According to Tantra, change is natural to the human self, the body-mind. But also according to Tantra, there is a changeless Self, which never changes, to which the changing self wakes up, discovers, embraces, and is absorbed into through transformative expansion. Thus there is both transformation and no-transformation. Change and no-change. According to Tantric Yoga the spiritual realm is the one changeless Being, or Brahma. This changeless realm, this Brahma, from which everything originates, from which everything is preserved and from within which everything dies and is destroyed, consists of two polarities: Shiva (Consciousness) and Shakti (Energy).

Shiva is that aspect of Brahma which is changeless, pure, subtle, the deep within, the deep inner world of all manifest beings, the deep inner space of the outer world, of matter, of the atomic world and beyond.

Shiva is pure consciousness, pure intelligence, from which even some quantum physicists now believe everything originates. Shiva is that oceanic space within, that cave in the cosmic heart, that which we experience while deep-diving the conscious and sub-conscious monkey-minds and enter the super-conscious mind of revelation and peace in our meditation.

In other words, in order to be awed by and to experience the inner thrill of Shiva Consciousness, we undergo a shift in aware-ness, an inner transformation with the help of Shakti energy, with the help of our will power, our emotions, and our physical energy. Because Shakti is pure energy, that which creates, that which binds consciousness into form, into life, creativity and finally into death. By riding the energy of Shakti, the kundalini of transformation and creativity, we embrace Shiva, the Changeless.

"Tantra is the process of transforming one's latent divinity into Supreme Divinity. A person who, irrespective of caste, creed or religion aspires for [such] spiritual expansion...is a Tantric." (Anan-damurtii, 1993)

Tantric yoga teaches us that if this unchanging reality, this Shiva is close to our heart, close to our inner mind in daily con-templation, in daily practice, then it is much easier to accept and welcome and challenge the turbulence of change—the pain of physical and mental suffering that also is an inevitable part of life. Hence, Tantra is to live in the balance of these two realms. By meditating on that Changeless Entity, that deep inner space of the cosmos, we embrace change, we accept change, we thrive on change in the form of Shakti, the goddess of transformation, creativity, destruction, and death.

By meditating on that Changeless Entity, we associate with the wave of breath that is always connected to the deep spiritual ocean within. And we come to realize, from experience, that when we are less agitated, angry, or irritated, that both Shiva (the changeless) and Shakti (that which always changes), these twin archetypes, are always alive within us.

Through continuous practice of Tantra, we begin to realize that when death strikes, when sickness strikes, that change is inevitable. We realize that it is Shakti's nature to change form, to transform, but that Shiva always remains formless and deeply whole within and beyond. We begin to realize that beyond duality there is nonduality. We realize that beyond both the deep subjective I of consciousness and the objective body—which may be healthy one day and sick the next—that beyond those polarities of our being, there is only Brahma, only Consciousness.

So, what is Tantric yoga, Tantric meditation? To shift our attention toward Shiva, toward Purusha, toward Consciousness, by embracing the energy of Shakti, the energy of Prakriti, the energy of transformation and change.

Shiva in us never changes, but the Shakti energy in us always undergoes transformation. And it thus is our choice to either use our Shakti energy wisely or to use it destructively. In other words, the practice of yoga is to use our Shakti energy wisely. We thus meditate in order to go beyond distraction and destruction and to experience wholeness and unity. We meditate to daily experience the subtle, changeless aspects of our soul, of our spirit.

"Ecstatic devotion to the Divine Mother [Shakti] alternated with serene absorption in the ocean of Absolute Unity [Shiva]. He thus bridged the gulf between the personal and impersonal, the immanent and transcendent aspects of reality."

—Swami Nikhilananda describing the Tantric spirituality of Shrii Ramakrishna

And here's the secret, the beauty of this transformation: by becoming more like the changeless, we can constantly undergo change more gracefully. We embrace change in the form of pain and suffering and joy more peacefully.

In other words, we do change, we do transform when we perform spiritual practice. Otherwise why bother to practice or to read and be moved by the great spiritual masterpieces, such as the Bhagavadgita? Otherwise why practice sense withdrawal, breathing exercises, mindfulness and ethics if not to gracefully transform that in us which needs to undergo change so that we can be awestruck by the changeless?

We do the practice, the asanas, the deep breathing, the counting of beads, the mantra repetition, to calm down the choppy winds of the mind, so that we may move into silence, flow toward the breath within the breath, toward the changeless nature of Spirit, toward Shiva, that unfathomable void that never undergoes any change.

We do this practice, sometimes painfully, other times boringly, but with steady diligence, our meditations become graceful and peaceful. We do this practice to generate change, to facilitate awakening. And gradually, we are transformed by this arousal of Shakti energy in our body and in our mind. In time, we are changed by it, except that part of us, that inner witness, that Shiva, that great cosmic I, that nondual awareness which never undergoes any change; that quiet breath within our breath, that witnessing I, deep within the quiet hurricane of our life.

Three Ways to Practice Yoga

Do you practice yoga to have` a flexible body, a bendable brain, an enlightened spirit, or to achieve a little bit of everything? Either way, you are not the first. Yoga has experimented with all these paths and expressions for centuries. But while looking at nearly twenty years of cover photos on a popular yoga magazine recently, it seemed as if modern yoga practice is primarily designed for the body, for outer appearance, fitness and flexibility. It also appeared as if yoga is primarily designed for perfectly shaped white women. Quite strikingly, the covers illustrated that a radical change took place some time in the late nineties.

Prior to that time, the magazine covers were artsy, the content often philosophical. But from then onward, the covers featured only attractive women with serene yoga-smiles and bodies exuding a wholesome allure. Still, the increasing popularity of yoga, in all its profane and divine manifestations, is a healthy and welcoming sign. As a young female yoga teacher told me: "I came to the deeper understanding of yoga by starting out thinking that yoga was only about physical flexibility." She quickly learned that yoga was so much more. She learned that yoga was about flexible bodies and flexible minds moving together, moving together toward Spirit.

As Pantanjali wrote in one of his famous yoga sutras, the goal of yoga is "the cessation of mental propensities." But in reading his text, we will not find any information about perfect anatomical alignment or sculpted hips. Patanjali's main focus remained way beyond bone and flesh, and to enable people to reach this goal of spiritual tranquility, he systematized Ashtanga Yoga based on already known yogic and Tantric wisdom practices.

In Patanjali's comprehensive system, yoga postures, or *asanas*, forms only one of eight parts: *yama* and *niyama* (ethics), *asanas* (yoga exercises), *pratyahara* (sense withdrawal), *dharana* (concentration), *pranayama* (breathing exercises), *dhyana* (meditation) and *samadhi* (spiritual peace). This system, often termed Classical Yoga by Western yoga scholars, built upon much earlier forms of yoga, including Samkhya philosophy, Tantric (Shaiva) meditation practices, and also, but to a much lesser degree, on the Vedas.

The goal of yoga, said Patanjali, is not just to attain control of the body, but rather to tame the mind. The final spiritual goal of yoga, he said, is reached when the mind is free of thoughts, desires and needs. While Patanjali's philosophy was dualistic—he did not as in the creation philosophy of Shaivism, or Tantra, explicitly unite the cosmic consciousness of Shiva and the cosmic energy of Shakti in the cosmic womb of nondual Brahma. But he did mention Ishvara, the cosmic Godhood, and he said that the goal of yoga was to experience Ishvara. After all, the tenth and last practice of yoga ethics, as per Patanjali, is Ishvara Pranidhana, the practice of meditating on Ishvara, on the Divine.

Metaphorically, the dualistic opposites of Shiva and Shakti are two sides of the same androgynous being; two dualistic sides of the nondual oneness of Brahma. And they were figuratively expressed in ancient art in the androgynous Ardhanarishvara statue, which according to Anandamurtii became a widespread idol and philosophical concept in Indian culture about 2500 years ago.

This ancient Tantric concept of yogic androgyny appeals to our contemporary, ecological sensibilities: everything is one, everything is interconnected. Where there is energy, there is consciousness. Where there is consciousness, there is energy. In Tantra, the goal of yoga is explicitly both Spirit-centered and body-centered. Because Shiva and Shakti are one. Tantric Yoga is therefore a practice of both earthly balance and spiritual union.

First a Tantric yogi attempts to harmonize body and mind, then to live in harmony with the world. Ultimately, he or she seeks *samadhi*, or spiritual union—the union between the human soul, or *jivatman*, and the Cosmic Soul, or *paramatman*. But that has not always been the case throughout yoga history. Not all yogis have viewed the body in the same positive light as Tantra.

Indeed, many famous modern yogis, including Vivekananda, did not think much of Hatha Yoga, or posture yoga, at all. This body-negation has been common in India since ancient times and is, in part, due to the influence of Vedanta, which viewed the body and the world as an illusion. In other words, yoga has expressed itself in different ways throughout the centuries; some forms viewed the body as divine, others as an illusion, or even sinful.

Ecstatic dancing and spiritual longing were also integral parts of some forms of yoga, most notably Tantric Bhakti Yoga. Today, these timeless expressions are bursting out of yoga studios, where kirtan artists such as Jai Uttal, Krishna Das and Wah! combine the sacredly inward with the beat-savvy outward rhythms of both East and West.

With the help of poets and translators like Coleman Barks, the medieval mystic Rumi is now a bestselling poet among yogis in

America. These are expressions of yoga practitioners' deep search for magic, ecstasy and otherworldly love. Meditation practice and classes on yoga ethics are also becoming an integral part of an increasing number of yoga teachers' offerings. Yes, in many yoga studios flexible bodies and flexible minds are fusing into spiritual union and oneness.

But in studios where there is a clear focus on yoga as a fitness exercise, kirtan artists are generally not invited. As mentioned before, this type of body-focused posture yoga has its roots in the tradition developed about a hundred years ago by Krishnamacarya, who mixed ancient yoga with modern gymnastics. This new Hatha Yoga tradition, in which meditation plays a minimal or non-existent part, has exploded in popularity and multiplicity in recent years in the US and Europe.

The goal of yoga's physical exercises in Tantra, on the other hand, was to create a healthy body and mind and thus a conducive environment for spiritual practice—for meditation. The physical exercises are part of a nested continuum, from body to mind to spirit. That's why, of course, it was emphasized in the Hatha Yoga Pradipika that Raja Yoga and Hatha Yoga should be practiced hand in hand.

And that is perhaps why B. K. S. Iyengar, the modern Hatha Yoga master par excellence, said in an online video that he wished he had started to meditate when he was younger, not at sixty-plus. The body is thus a springboard from which a self-inspired and sustainable spirit can soar. Many of the fitness yogis and yoginis of today may not see it the same way. For them, a beautiful, healthy body and an alert mind is more likely the main goal.

In other words, if yoga makes me more flexible, more relaxed, more beautiful, so that I can be more efficient, more powerful, more attractive, why ask for more? Why ask for more, if the body simply is a springboard from which a dazzlingly successful me will ascend? Many of the yogis of old, however, did indeed ask for more. The intertwined distinctions they made between body, mind and spirit is a brilliant insight of yoga practice and philosophy.

Yoga teaches us that any improvement on the physical or mental level can never be perfect, can never be ultimately fulfilling, and will always leave us shortchanged. Truth is, that perfect body will never quite be perfect enough. But, truth be also told, some yogis of old were as extremely body-negative as many of today's yogis are extreme in their hedonistic body positivity. In other words, there is a lack of ecology, of balance in each of these approaches, in the cult of the *Yoga Journal* body-sculpting women as well as in the body-negating cult of yogis who deny the body through their display of atrophying arms or legs.

Tantra has attempted a different approach, and has often walked that fine balance beautifully by embracing both body and soul, both Shakti and Shiva, both *Prakriti* and *Purusha*, both the inner and outer world. The physical realm of our existence is indeed limited. The body will finally age. It may start to ache. Disease may come. Thus, "I am not this body," the spiritual yogi would say. "I am not this mind. I am That. I am divine."

Behind the sensuous gloss on the covers of today's yoga magazines, we do see some glimpses of the deeper, subterranean flow of yogic wisdom and practice. In yoga studios all over the world, harmoniums and tablas are placed before outstretched yoga mats. Some are even dusting off the Bhagavad Gita's urging that we practice karma yoga, selfless service or social change activities. Ayurvedic massage and herbs are integral healing modalities in many yoga studios. Many yoga teachers end their classes with at least rudimentary forms of meditation. These are all signs of a holistic tapestry being woven together from all the integrated strands of wisdom yoga can offer.

Keeping this perspective in our mind, like a silent mantra behind silent lips, we can stay more balanced, more honest, more authentically yogi-like—both on and off the mat. As Sufi poet Rumi says, it is indeed important to know what you want. Because, says this wise poet of ecstasy: "There is a subtle truth: whatever you love, you are."

Three Ways to Yogic Enlightenment

In reality, there are many more, perhaps as many as there are yogis, but just for the sake of limited space and the topic of this book, I will introduce three distinct and influential philosophical paths within traditional yoga philosophy. While doing so, we will look at each philosophy's unique way to uncover the essence of yoga, which, according to Michael Stone, author of the insightful and very readable *The Inner Tradition of Yoga*, is simply this: to teach us "that all forms of clinging create suffering." (Stone, 2008)

However, while all paths of yoga teaches us about the futility of attachments to our ego: the way our body looks, how much money we make, how big or small our nose is, etc., not all paths of yoga puts so much emphasis on the avoidance of attachment and of suffering. Buddha said that suffering exists; it has a cause; it has an end; and it has a cause to bring about its end. While Buddhism emphasizes suffering, Tantra instructs us that the practice of yoga reveals feelings of joy, freedom, wholeness, bliss, love, awe, expansion, oneness. Krishna's sublime stories in the Bhagavadgita are also about a different mind-set: to see all as love, embrace all as sacred, see all as one.

A yogi, whose life's goal is to end suffering, achieves enlightenment through detachment leading to transcendental absorption. This path of discernment, this path of calm, focused discrimination is different from the path of celebratory union, the path of sacred embrace as emphasized in the heart-centered Bhakti Yoga of Kabir, or the ecstatic Kali-worshiping Tantra of Ramakrishna. Yet, as we will see, all yogic paths are intertwined like threads in a meditation rug. They have much more in common than not. And it is this Tantric commonality which holds the promise of a yogic future embracing the spirit of unity in diversity.

Brief outline of three traditional paths
of yogic enlightenment:

Patanjali's Yoga, or *dvaita*; traditionally considered a dualist school of yoga.

Adi Shankara's Vedanta, or *advaita*; traditionally considered nondualist, or *mayavada* (the doctrine of illusion/only Brahma/God is real).

Tantra, or *advaita-dvaita-advaita*; traditionally nondualist; but more appropriately a nondualistic-dualistic-nondualist philosophy bridging the philosophical dichotomy between Patanjali Yoga and Vedanta.

Patanjali Yoga and Tantra

The Classical Yoga of Patanjali is in traditional India also referred to as Patanjali Samkhya, Patanjali Tantra, or Raja Yoga. This is not accidental. When referred to as Samkhya, it is because Patanjali's Yoga Sutras follow and expand upon the tradition of the incredibly sophisticated philosophy of Kapila's Samkhya, which is also the philosophical foundation of Ayurveda, India's yoga-based medical system. Hence, to deeply understand the principles of both Ayurveda and yoga, studying the detailed and logical cosmology of Samkhya philosophy is exceedingly instructive.

Samkhya is also sometimes referred to as Kapilasya Tantra, after its founder Kapila, to indicate its link to early Shaiva Tantra. Samkhya is also termed Tantra Shaivism, and Ayurveda is also characterized as "Tantric medicine," or "Siddha medicine," especially in East and South India. In other words, while there are distinct differences between these important schools and practices, there are many more integrating similarities. While Patanjali followed in the footsteps of Kapila, he again built upon the works of the ancient Vedic and Tantric (Shaiva) sages of the past. Most all of the meditation teachings outlined in the Yoga Sutras, for example, are practiced widely among all yogic traditions.

Likewise, Shankara was a Shiva Tantric and presumed to be the founder of Vedanta (Feuerstein, 2001, Anandamurtii, 1993) who followed in the footsteps of Patanjali, and the Tantric sages of the middle ages, those half-naked sadhus who penned the various textbooks on Hatha Yoga. But, in true Indian tradition, he advanced his own philosophical school, and he was known as a fierce debater and logician, often debating Buddhist monks.

The Natha Tantrics of the Middle Ages, who wrote the Hatha Yoga texts dedicated to Shiva, followed in the footsteps of an old oral tradition in part recorded in the Puranas, the Upanishads, the Bhagavad Gita,the Tantras, the Agamas, and the Shiva Samhitas. These yogis hailed from a fertile Tantric tradition that in many ways was distinctly non-Vedic. This potpourri of ideas and practices spawned a plethora of philosophical sub-schools and traditions with names and founders, practices, myths and meanings as numerous and colorful as the patterns in an Indian sari, but according to Anandamurtii, all these schools are Tantric in view of their essential spiritual practices.

Let us take a brief look at these three schools:

Patanjali's Yoga Sutras

Patanjali's philosophy (approximately 200 BCE) recognizes the Self (Purusha) as a transcendental, all-pervading entity and as a state of mind actualized by a self-realized yogi. The opposite reality of the Self is the World (Prakrti) with all its numerous physical and mental manifestations. The yogi's delusion according to Patanjali is the preoccupation with the world, the senses, the body, etc.

Thus, in his dualistic view of realty, Patanjali encourages the yogi, by following the eight limbs of yoga, to disengage and withdraw from the world through ethical behavior, study, postures, breathing exercises and meditation to reach samadhi, the final absorption in the Self. The false identification with the world is the allure that draws the yogi away from the inner world of the one true Self.

Patanjali did not promote union with the Self through longing and heart-centered worship or meditation as in Bhakti or Tantra Yoga. Rather his way to liberation and enlightenment is to escape suffering via discernment, introspection, and meditation. Patanjali draws a distinct separation between the Self and the non-self; it is evidently not a yoga of union. This is how yoga scholar Georg Feuerstein reads him: "Given Patanjali's dualist metaphysics, which strictly separates the transcendental Self from Nature and its products, [union] would not even make any sense." (Feuerstein, 1989)

For yoga philosopher and psychologist Michael Stone, we have lost nothing and gained everything with such an attitude. Yoga, according to Stone, is not an act of unity. This turns yoga into a "willful activity," he writes; quite the opposite of what Patanjali intended. Yoga, according to Stone, "means that everything is interdependent…not something we seek outside ourselves or a willful attempt at union, but the recognition, in the present moment, of the unification of life."

A yogi on Patanjali's path gradually discover a deeper recognition of the inner Self, and eventually realizes, through skillful separation of truth from untruth, the nondual awareness of the transcendental reality. Hence, the path of duality, artfully practiced, leads to nonduality and enlightenment. This process toward enlightenment according to Patanjali does not occur through union, but as a process of shifting our identity, of identifying with the transcendental rather than with the worldly.

The strength and beauty of Patanjali's Yoga Sutras lies, I think, in his insightful gifts of philosophical detail on the path of discerning what the Self is not. Moreover, the Yoga Sutras' contemplative stanzas and practical insights about meditation are an integral part of many yogis' daily practices both on and off the cushion and mat. The Yoga Sutras are not an instruction manual in meditation, however. A competent teacher who can impart the practical lessons of *pranayama* (breathing exercises), *pratyahara* (sense withdrawal) *dharana* (concentration) and *dhyana* (focused flow) is thus essential in order to develop a daily, personal meditation practice.

Advaita Vedanta

Shankara, or Shankaracharya (approximately 800 CE), was a Shaiva Tantrika, or practioner of Tantra who, like many Indian ascetics, was a follower Shiva. He believed in Nirguna Brahma, or Purusha only. His theories are reminiscent of *shunyavada* in Buddhism, the doctrine of emptiness. Unlike Patanjali, he did not believe in the existence of *jagat*, or the physical world, and he promoted Gunanvita Mayavada, the doctrine of illusion.

Shankara's doctrine was summed up in the following sutra:

Brahma satyam jagat mithya, jivo brahmaiva na parah

Brahma is the only truth, the spatial-temporal world is an illusion, and there is ultimately no difference between Brahma and the individual self.

Shankara was a great logician and traveled throughout India teaching his new doctrine. During his short, thirty-two-year-old life, he managed to unite the various Hindu sects and to greatly reduce the influence of Buddhism in India. Because of his philosophical unification of two seemingly disparate philosophical concepts, *atman* (individual self) and Brahma, many think of him as the most brilliant philosopher, a kind of St. Thomas of Aquinas, in the history of Indian thought.

As a Tantric yogi, Shankara taught the practices of kundalini yoga and the esoteric science of mantra meditation. In Swami Vivekananada (1863-1902) we witness a modern exponent of Vedanta and simultaneously a teacher following the eight-fold path of Patanjali's Yoga Sutras, or Raja Yoga. Moreover, Vivekananda, was an ardent social reformer and not exactly one to act as if the world was an illusion.

Shankara's doctrine of illusion undoubtedly has had many negative social effects in India by enslaving people to fatalist dogmas steeped in caste, myth and oppression. Yet, in giant personalities like Vivekananda and Aurobindu (1872-1950), both greatly influenced by Patanjali and Shankara, we witness a modern integration reconciling the deep spiritual introspection of yogic India with western Enlightenment rationality and social reform.

In other words, we see in Vivekananda and Aurobindu a fruitful integration of the dualism of Patanjali with the non-dualism of Shankara. Quite tellingly, Aurobindu called his yoga Integral Yoga and Georg Feuerstein thinks it is Aurobindo, more than any other yogi, who epitomizes the birth of modern yoga in the world. The millions of "posture yogis" in the West would perhaps disagree and instead think of Krishnamacharya as a more likely candidate. Others would contend that it is Anandamurtii who represents the holistic future of yoga as he has revived the ancient Tantra practices for the modern age, developed a new and comprehensive Tantric cosmology, thereby uniting the duality of Samkhya and Patanjali with the nonduality of Vedanta.

Tantra

If the Vedanta of Vivekananda, or Deepak Chopra—who makes a point about not being a Hindu but rather a follower of Vedanta—signifies the modern version of ancient yoga, it is perhaps Tantra, more than any other form of yogic philosophy, that embody a post-modern and integral vision.

Philosopher Ken Wilber maintains that the nondualism of Tantra brings together the inseparable and eternal unity of Purusha and Prakrti in a "nondual embrace" of fundamental importance to yogic philosophy. This logical embrace reconciles the best of Patanjali with the best of Shankara, the essence of dualism with the essence of nondualism. (Wilber, 2001) No other modern Tantra philosopher has expressed this nondual embrace better than Anandamurtii, I think, whose book Ananda Sutram creates perhaps the fullest, nondual synthesis of any Tantric or yogic text so far produced.

As philosophy, the ancient, oral tradition of Tantra is a relative late-comer in India and is associated with the "Tantric Renaissance" of the Middle Ages, when almost all of the Tantric texts dedicated to Shiva—its alleged originator and King of Yoga—were authored. According to Feuerstein, "By unifying the mind—that is, by focusing it—Tantra Yoga unifies the seemingly disparate realities of space-time and the transcendental Reality." (Feuerstein, 1998) In other words, Tantra beautifully unifies the duality of Patanjali with the nonduality of Vedanta.

Tantra bridges the contradictions between Vedanta's the-world-is-an-illusion theory with Patanajali's the-world-is-a-distraction philosophy by exclaiming that both the world and Spirit are Brahma, and that all THIS is real. Tantra, like Krishna in the Gita, instructs us: I am That, I am always unified with That. I am Consciousness, and Consciousness made the world. Hence the use of will, the practice of observation, discernment, love, are not at all contradictory to Tantra. Each aspect of reality complements each other in a cosmic embrace of spiritual union. Purusha and Prakrti, these universal opposites of Spirit and flesh are truly one in Brahma, truly two aspects of the same Transcendental Consciousness.

The biggest challenge for the followers of Vedanta is perhaps to avoid confusing the intellectual understanding of nonduality with the actual experience of it. To free oneself from the idea that "I am enlightened just because I think I am." The challenge for the dualist, on the other hand, is to let go of the mind and also to perceive the world openly through the heart. For Tantra, perhaps the biggest challenge is the idea that, since Spirit is everywhere, therefore anything goes; therefore any behavior is spiritual behavior; therefore, as we see in so many neo-Tantric circles, the flesh is hedonistically mistaken for Spirit, and indulgence equals transcendence.

A Common Philosophical Weave

In truth, I think we can learn from, and integrate, all of these philosophical yogic paths into our own. Dualism is part of realizing non-dualism. Without a body, without experiencing separation and longing, we cannot practice the yoga of nondualism in the first place. Thus all three yogic paths can be balanced and interconnected.

Although I personally favor Tantra—for Tantra is the practical and yogic core of all these three paths, this impossibly tongue-tied philosophical vision we may call nondualistic-dualistic-nondualism—I humbly bow to the rich inner wisdom of all three paths.

In summary, we exist in this world. We are not an illusion. Nor is the world an illusion, nor does it have to be a trap of the flesh. Both we and the world are physically and spiritually vibrant, real and present in all our glory. All of the time. Yet, when we are trapped in the world, we mistake the unreal for the real, the rope for a snake, and life's lessons do indeed become fleeting and illusory.

The inner spirit of these three paths to enlightenment is perhaps most beautifully summed up in the koan-like words of the great nondual sage Ramana Maharishi, who traditionally is referred to as a Vedantic sage, but who also was a follower of Shiva, the original Adi-yogi, the Tantric King of Yoga:

The world is illusory;
Brahma alone is real;
Brahma is the world.

This idea, that the world is spirit, that the world is sacred, is one of Tantra's many gifts to humanity. In this profoundly simple concept, that the Divine is both within and outside us, lies the secret essence of yoga and to all mystic spirituality at the heart of all religions. The future of yoga, therefore, lies not simply in its current proliferation and popularity of yoga poses for better health, but rather in returning to its ancient roots, to its holistic nature, to the perennial Tantric quest, since the beginning of historical time: the eternal search for vibrant physical health, an awakened mind and a transcendent spirit.

Bibliography

Abhayananda, S., *The History of Mysticism*, ATMA Books, Olympia, Washington, 1998

Avalon, Arthur, (Sir John Woodroffe), *The Serpent Power*, Dover Publications, New York, 1974

Anandamitra, Acarya, *The Spiritual Philosophy of Shrii Shrii Anandamurtii: A Commentary on Ananda Sutram*, Ananda Marga Publications, Kolkata, 1998Anandamurtii, Shrii Shrii, *Discourses on Tantra, Volume 2*, Ananda Marga Publications, Kolkata, 1994

Ibid., *Discourses on Tantra, Volume I*, Ananda Marga Publications, Kolkata, 1994

Ibid., *Yoga Sadhana: The Spiritual Practice of Yoga*, Ananda Marga Publications, Kolkata, 2010

Ibid., *Namah Shivaya Shantaya*, Ananda Marga Publications, Kolkata, 1993

Bhattacharyya, N. N., *The History of the Tantric Religion*, Manohar Publishing, New Delhi

Bhamshad, Michael J., http://jorde-lab.genetics.utah.edu/elibrary/Bamshad_2001a.pdf

Bjonnes, Ramesh, *Tantra: The Yoga of Love and Awakening*, Hay House, New Delhi, India, 2014

Ibid, *Tantra and Veda: The Untold Story*, article published on www.integralworld.net

Ibid, *Sacred Body, Sacred Spirit*, Innerworld Publications, 2012

Bly, Robert, *The Soul is Here for Its Own Joy*, Ecco Press, 1999

Cooke, Robert, *History of Aryan Conquest of India told in Genes*, San Francisco Chronicle, 26 May, 1999

Crow, David, *In Search of the Medicine Buddha*, Tarcher/Putnam, New York, 2000

Danielou, Alain, *While the Gods Play*, Inner Traditions, Rochester, Vermont, 1987

Ibid., *A Brief History of India*, Inner Traditions, Rochester, Vermont, 1994

Ibid., *Shiva and the Primordial Tradition*, Inner Tradition, Rochester, Vermont, 2006

Feuerstein, Georg, *The Yoga Tradition*, Hohm Press, Chino Valley, 2001

Ibid., *Tantra: The Path of Ecstasy*, Shambhala, Boston, 1998

Ibid., *In Search of the Cradle of Human Civilization*, Quest Books, Wheaton, IL, 1995

Ibid., *The Yoga-Sutra of Patanjali*, Inner Traditions, Vermont, 1989

Goswami, Shyam Sundar, *Laya Yoga: The Definitive Guide to the Chakras and Kundalini*, Inner Tradition, Vermont, 1999

Hensberger, Beth, *The Ultimate Rice Cooker Cookbook*, Harvard Common Press, 2002

Hixon, Lex, *Coming Home*, Larson Publications, 1995

Hunter, Dennis, quote from his website www.dennishuntermeditation.com

Kumar, Arvin, *Women and the Vedas: Limiting Women Limits All of Society*, *India Currents*, September, 1994

Marshall, Sir John, *Mohenjo-Daro and The Indus Valley Civilization*, Asian Educational Services, 1931

Manoharan, S, *Peopling Of India*, Independent research paper published by Madhav Gadgil, N. V. Joshi from Indian Institute of Science; U. V. Shambu Prasad, Centre for Research in Indo-Bangladesh Relations; S. Manoharan and Suresh Patil from Anthropological Survey of India. http://ces.iisc.ernet.in/hpg/cesmg/peopling.html#sec1

Muller, Max, *The Veda: Chips from a German Workshop*, vol 1, New York, Charles Scribner, 1900, p. 63

McEvilley, Thomas, *An Archeology of Yoga*, Anthropology and Aesthetics, 1981

Neale, Miles, *Frozen Yoga and McMindfulness*, an interview published in Lion's Roar, December 15, 2010

Oma Armstrong, Kristin, *Yoga in the Bronze Age?*, essay in *Facets of Archeology*, Oslo, 2008

Roche, Lorin, *The Radiance Sutras*, Sounds True, Boulder, CO, 2016

Singh, Lalan Prasad, *Tantra: Its Mystic and Scientific Basis*, Concept Publishing, New Delhi, 1976

Satyananda, Swami, *Kundalini Tantra*, Yoga Publications Trust, Bihar, India, 1984

Sakhare, M.R., *History and Philosophy of the Lingayat Religion*, Karnatak University, 1978

Sidharth, B. G., *The Celestial Key to the Vedas*, Inner Traditions International, Vermont, 1999

Steindl-Rast, David, *Belonging to the Universe*, Harper, San Francisco, 1992

Stone, Michael, *The Inner Tradition of Yoga*, Shambala Publications, 2008

McEvilley, Thomas, *An Archeology of Yoga*, University of Chicago Press Journals, 1981

Mallinson, James and Singleton, Mark, *The Roots of Yoga: The Origin of Modern Posture Yoga*, Penguin Classics, UK, 2017

McClure, Vimala, *A Woman's Guide to Tantra Yoga*, New World Library, 1997

Wallis, Christopher, *Tantra Illuminated*, Mattamayura Press, Petaluma, 2012

Wells, Spencer, *The Journey of Man: A Genetic Odyssey*, Princeton Science Library, Princeton, NJ, 2017

Wilber, Ken, *Sex, Ecology, Spirituality*, Shambala, Boston, 1996

Wolf-Dieter, Storl, *Shiva: The Wild God Of Ecstasy*, Inner Traditions, Vermont, 2004, page 178

Woodroffe, John, *Principles of Tantra, Part II*, Ganesh and Co, Madras, 1970

Ibid., Interview with Dr. Spencer Wells, www.rediff.com http://www.rediff.com/news/2002/nov/27inter.htm   November, 2002

Wright, Robert, *Why Buddhism is True: The Science and Philosophy of Meditation and Enlightenment*, Simon and Schuster, New York, 2018

Glossary

AGAMA AND NIGAMA: Agama is the applied or practical side of Tantra and Nigama is the theoretical side. In Tantric texts, NIGAMA also represent the questions asked by PARVATI to SHIVA and AGAMA represent his answers.

ASTHANGA YOGA: The eight-limbed path of yoga systematized by Patanjali in the Yoga Sutras, a text dated to about 200 BCE.

ANANDA SUTRAM: Literally "aphorisms leading to Bliss," following in the tradition of Kapila's Samkhya and Patanjali's Yoga Sutras, Ananda Sutram comprises eighty five sutras of Shrii Shrii Anandamurti's Tantric philosophy and cosmology.

ATHARVAVEDA: One of the ancient four Vedic texts most influenced by Tantra.

ATMAN: Soul, consciousness. The Atman of the cosmos is Paramatman, while the atman of human beings is termed Jivatman.

AVIDYA SHAKTI: the force which propels us away from wisdom toward ignorance and from the subtle toward the crude.

AYURVEDA: the yogic or Tantric system of natural medicine using herbs, food, yoga, and meditation to heal.

BHAGAVAD GITA: "Song of God." The sacred text which contains Krishna's spiritual advice to Arjuna on the battlefield, just before the Mahabharata war.

BHAKTI: devotion.

BHAKTI YOGA: Devotional form of spiritual practice, such as chanting, prayer, dancing, singing, etc.

BRAHMA: Cosmic Consciousness, comprising both PURUSHA, or SHIVA, and PRAKRTI, or SHAKTI.

BRAHMAN: a high caste person who traditionally perform priestly functions or live by intellectual labor.

CHAKRA: literally "cycle or circle;" a psycho-spiritual center or plexus in the body as part of the subtle body in Tantra. The seven main chakras are located along the *susumna* channel which passes through the spinal column and extends to the crown of the head. In Tantra, chakras are associated with external concentration points and used in meditation combined with mantras and visualization techniques. The chakras are also related to the *vrittis*, various mental and emotional expressions located in the chakras, which again are related to the human endocrine glands, as well as the nervous system.

CITTA: the mind, sometimes referred to as heart-mind, the emotional and mental mind.

DEVA: Mythological being, a god, a deity.

DEVI: A goddess, a female deity.

DHARANA: The sixth limb of Asthanga Yoga; concentration on particular points in the body, or chakras, using mantra and/or various visualization techniques.

DHARMA: The natural characteristic of something; the path of spirituality; righteousness in social affairs.

DHYANA: Seventh limb of Asthanga Yoga; meditation technique in which the mind is directed in one flow towards Cosmic Consciousness, towards BRAHMA; an advanced visualization practice in Tantra in which the goal is to merge in Cosmic Consciousness.

GUNA: attribute of nature; PRAKRTI; in Tantric cosmology, the Cosmic Energy Principle, or Cosmic Operative Principle is composed of: sattvaguna, the peaceful principle; rajaguna, the energetic principle; and tamaguna, the static principle.

GURU: Literally "dispeller of darkness;" a self-realized master of Tantra and yoga; a MAHAKAOLA; one who can raise the KUNDALINI of others; one who initiates others on the path of Tantra by imparting a SIDDHA MANTRA. Throughout history there has only been a small group of self-realized beings at any given time, people who, in the tradition of yoga, truly deserve the title GURU. Therefore, many so-called gurus are not self-realized masters, but rather people with flawed character traits; thus the controversial nature of the term.

ISHVARA: God, the Cosmic Controller.

JAPA: Repetition of mantra.

JIVA: An individual being.

JIVATMAN: the soul of a human being.

JNANA: knowledge, understanding.

JNANA YOGA: spiritual practice aiming at self-realization through the path of knowledge.

KAOLA: one who practices *kula* meditation and is adept at raising his or her own KUNDALINI.

KAPALIKA(S): a Tantric yogi; a specific order of Tantric yogis.

KAPALIKA SADHANA: a specific Tantric meditation performed at night in cremation grounds to overcome all the inherent fetters of the human mind.

KARMA: Action; positive or negative actions which results in SAMSKARAS.

KARMA YOGA: A form of spiritual practice which aims at self-realization through the path of selfless action.

KIRTAN: Chanting of mantras, sometimes while dancing; the spirit of longing and feelings of devotion for God.

KSATTRIYA: High caste in the Vedic system, one who traditionally belonged to the military class.

KUNDALINI: Literally "coiled serpentine;" dormant divinity; the force in the *kula* (first chakra at the bottom of the spine) which, when awakened, rises up the spinal column, piercing through the various chakras and awakening one's innate spiritual potential.

MADHUVIDYA: Literally "honey knowledge;" the Tantric practice of seeing all objects, people, thoughts, feelings, and actions as an expression of BRAHMA, of Cosmic Consciousness, of the Divine.

MAHAKAOLA: A Tantric guru who can raise not only his own KUNDALINI but also that of others.

MANTRA: Literally "that which liberates the mind;" a word, or set of Sanskrit syllables which when meditated upon or chanted can arouse the KUNDALINI resulting in spiritual awakening, feelings of bliss and peace, and spiritual liberation. A Tantric mantra has three qualities: it is pulsative (it has two syllables corresponding to one's inhalation and exhalation), it is incantative (it enables one's individual vibration to be united with the cosmic vibration of consciousness) and it is ideative (it has a deep spiritual meaning).

MANTRA CAETANYA: The spiritual awakening caused by MANTRA meditation.

MAYA: Another name for PRAKRTI, or SHAKTI; the power of PRAKRTI to cause the illusion that the material world is the only truth.

MOKSHA: Spiritual liberation.

MUDRA: Spiritual gesture as part of Indian dance, or a hand gesture used by a Tantric master to evoke spiritual awakening.

NIRGUNA BRAHMA: The state of BRAHMA before creation, the state of pure Cosmic Consciousness in Tantric cosmology.

OM: The sound of the first expression of creation; the seed mantra of the entire expressed universe.

PARAMATMAN: Cosmic Consciousness in the role as witness to all of creation.

PRAKRTI: The Cosmic Energy Principle, or Cosmic Operative Principle, also termed SHAKTI; the cosmic force which creates nature.

PRANAYAMA: The fourth limb of Ashtanga Yoga; the process of meditation on the breath with or without the use of mantra; the process of controlling vital energy by controlling the breath.

PRATYAHARA: The fifth limb of Ashtanga Yoga; the meditation process of withdrawing the mind from absorption in the physical senses.

PURANA: A mythological story, or historical chronology.

SHIVA: The first Guru, or Adiguru, of Tantra; a historical personality at the dawn of human civilization who systematized Tantra into a comprehensive yogic science; the historical King of

Yoga; the principle of Cosmic Consciousness in Tantric cosmology; a God in the Hindu pantheon.

SADHANA: Literally "sustained effort;" spiritual practice, meditation.

SADHAKA: Spiritual practitioner.

SAMADHI: Absorption of the human mind into the psycho-spiritual or purely spiritual realm. There are various forms of Samadhi depending on the stage of one's spiritual awakening.

SAMKHYA: The ancient Tantric philosophy and cosmology of "enumeration" advanced by Kapila around 1500 BCE, which forms the basis of Ayurvedic philosophy, dualist Tantra, as well as Patanjali's Yoga sutras; also called Kapilasya Tantra.

SAMSKARA: Mental reaction based on past action in potential form.

SHAKTA: A follower of the path of Shakta Tantra, in which the force of SHAKTI is worshipped and used for spiritual growth.

SIDDHA MANTRA: A mantra perfected by a MAHAKAOLA, a GURU who knows the intuitional science of mantra.

SIDDHA MEDICINE: Tantric form of Ayurveda popular in South India.

SHAIVA TANTRA: The original, practical teachings of Tantra given by SHIVA; the historical tradition of Tantra.

SHAIVA DHARMA: All of SHIVA'S teachings, both practical and philosophical.

SHIVOKTI: The sayings of SHIVA.

SHIVOPADESHA: The practical instructions of SHIVA.

SHUDRA: The lowest caste in the Vedic system; one who lives by manual labor.

TANTRA: A spiritual tradition which originated with the teachings of SHIVA; the original source of yoga. Also, a scripture expounding the tradition.

VAEDYAK SHASTRA: The Ayurvedic school of medicine developed by SHIVA.

VEDA: Literally "knowledge;" a religious or philosophical school which originated with the Vedic Aryans; a religious tradition emphasizing the use of ritual to gain the intervention of the gods. There are four main Vedas—the Rigveda, the Atharvaveda, the Samaveda and the Yajurveda. There is also a so-called Fifth Veda comprising the Upanishads, the Bhagavadgita and the Brahmanas, the ancient, oral teachings of the yogis written down as texts from around 800 BCE onwards. When scholars speak or write about Vedic philosophy, they generally refer to the Fifth Veda, which was highly influenced by Tantra and the practices of Tantric yogis.

VIDYA: Literally "knowledge;" the Cosmic Force of wisdom guiding us toward the path of spirituality.

VRITTI: Mental propensity; desire; instinct.

YAJNA: Vedic ritual offering.

YOGA: Spiritual practice of meditation leading to union between the human soul (Jivatman) and the cosmic soul (Paramatman); the practice of various postures and meditation techniques for health and spiritual growth. In reality, the paths of Tantra and yoga are similar; even synonymous.

CPSIA information can be obtained
at www.ICGtesting.com
Printed in the USA
LVHW111646190821
695554LV00003B/503

9 781881 717638